WESTEI

& CHINESE MEDICINE

Examines the many theoretical and practical interactions between astrology in the West and traditional Chinese medicine.

WESTERN ASTROLOGY & CHINESE MEDICINE

by

JONATHAN CLOGSTOUN-WILLMOTT

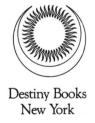

Destiny Books
New York

Destiny Books
377 Park Avenue South
New York, NY 10016

First quality paperback edition: August 1985

10 9 8 7 6 5 4 3 2 1

ISBN 0 89281 109 9

Destiny Books is a division of Inner Traditions International, Ltd.

Printed and bound in Great Britain

CONTENTS

ACKNOWLEDGEMENTS

Grateful thanks —

To Mary Austin for her inspiration and guidance.
To the doctors and colleagues I met in China, especially in Nanjing.
For the knowledge and wisdom of teachers and friends at many
seminars and courses, such as those given by Dr T. J. Kaptchuk, Dr
J. Shen, Professor J. Worsley, Penny Brohn, the Faculty of Astrological
Studies, Peter Holmes and many others.
To my editor for his patience.
To my patients for their forbearance.
To Sheila Cowperthwaite for drawing my doodles and typing my
scrawls.
To my wife Maureen for constructive criticism and for holding me
together.

Note: In all cases where the words *fire, earth* and *water* occur, they
refer to the Chinese medical phases, unless specifically stated.

INTRODUCTION

This book is not a description of astrology; I mention only certain aspects of each planet, and very little about how to interpret a chart. But non-astrologers and astrologers alike should be able to gain some insight into the thinking behind traditional Chinese medicine and how it views their health.

I have omitted not a few factors in traditional Chinese medicine which others may consider important, as this is an introductory work of limited space. Sadly also there is not much room for discussion of astrological transits and progressions.

Astrologers! Beware the temptation to predict disease from a chart! If an individual is alive, there is always hope for something better. An unguarded word can crush that hope. If possible, diagnose the state of health first; then use the chart to guide your patient to a deeper understanding and a broader perspective of his (or her) life, in the hope that by perceiving his place in the universe he may achieve healthy wholeness again. In all therapies, we have to try to imagine how the patient might be, devoid of hindrances. At times, planetary positions show us characteristic blocks that both define and limit; it is these that the astrologer must attempt to see beyond.

In this book, each planet is described as having a main function. It is a mistake to assume that two systems of thought — traditional Chinese medicine and Western astrology — will dovetail perfectly. All planets contain aspects of all energetic functions. Only the main emphasis is described here.

In the West, there is a tendency to confuse acupuncture with the totality of Chinese medicine. In China, acupuncture and herbalism are only two of the subjects that must be learnt, and each is, to some extent, a speciality. Herbalism is more difficult and takes longer. Some would say that it has a better reputation. But to traditional doctors, an effective treatment might comprise advice on just a small matter of diet and a particular Tai Qi movement: this might be sufficient for that patient. Westerners are harder to please. They want action and responsibility on the part of their therapist.

It is my belief that Chinese medicine and astrology are most useful when guiding individuals back towards an understanding of what they can do to help themselves, and in the case of Chinese medicine, intervening only when all else fails.

The views expressed about the relationship between traditional Chinese medicine and Western astrology are mine, and as I expect to alter some of them in due course, I welcome constructive criticism and opinions!

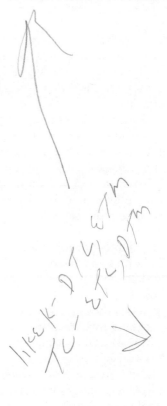

1.
THE CYCLES

The Principles of Traditional Chinese Medicine

The basic principle in traditional Chinese medicine is clear: pain is due to blockage in a flow of energy, too much or too little of it. If the blockage can be removed, the excess dispersed or the deficit resolved, the pain will disappear.

The practitioner of traditional Chinese medicine, if confronted by something he cannot comprehend, asks more questions until he does understand. He realizes how important his first action on an unstable energy system can be. Should he disperse energy or fortify it? Given that his patient expects so much, it may be well to get the direction of his effort right rather than risk disappointment. This is very different to the Western approach, which usually aims to alleviate pain as a first priority, no matter what the effect on the patient's vitality.

The Chinese are very pragmatic: if it works, use it. They would applaud any method that promotes health. They were quick to exploit electroacupuncture, especially in anaesthesia, and they cheerfully combine drug treatment with their endogenous system, where appropriate. They can do this because they can incorporate the effects of drugs into their philosophy more easily than we in the West can incorporate an unknown 'folk' medicine into our own system. Their system is built on very simple principles to which everything is related. Indeed, it has been said that one difference between oriental and Western medicine is that the latter takes many years to learn, but is comparatively easy to apply, whereas the former is easy to learn — there are fundamentally only two things to grasp — but difficult to apply, because those fundamental principles are applied in every case. This makes a good practitioner of traditional Chinese medicine very sure of himself philosophically, and often able, from the association of his medical pathology, to make quite accurate 'guesses' about his patient's background and life. Perhaps this is because he is used to looking for patterns of behaviour that incorporate both substance and psyche, both physical ailment and character.

This is good news to the astrologer! Someone else, for thousands of years, has been thinking the way that he does.

Medicine and Astrology

So the Chinese are pragmatic. Let us follow their example. Their own astrology, although splendid, is tied to their own culture. Our astrology is more accessible to us, is more sophisticated, and once gave useful service to doctors and herbalists, if only as a means of understanding their patients. Perhaps Western astrology can become still more useful when combined with the observations of character and disease made by Chinese over the millennia!

There are other similarities between the Western astrological view of life and that of the Chinese. In interpreting a chart we are, or should try to become, humble. We know that the horoscope does not describe the personality in its entirety. After all, it uses only eight planets, Sun and Moon. Only a chart that included everything in the whole universe could adequately define an individual, and, given nature's desire to explore, probably not even then. Even so, it is an astrologer's belief that the chart does show the flux of potential in life, and that if understood, each part is reflected in the whole, which would not be the same were the least part altered. Beneath this lies a basic insight shared with Chinese thought — that the least part of the picture, properly understood, shows the whole, just as a small fragment of glass or crystal in which a picture has been imprinted in holograph will, given the right source of light, show the whole again.

Put another way, a patient with a chronically septic finger betrays his personality to those who can perceive it in the same way as Mars in Gemini on the cusp of the 3rd house in a horoscope: it does of itself not give a whole picture, but the picture once seen must be consonant with it, no matter how illogical. Each part of the picture, rightly viewed, describes the whole. Astrologers are well prepared for their encounter with Chinese philosophy.

Another advantage of an astrological background is an awareness of what 'rulership' or 'association' means. An astrologer would never say (or *should* never say) that because his client has Sun in Leo, therefore his client's heart (Leo is astrologically associated with the heart organ, amongst other things) was in danger. (He might well talk about a lack of, or excess of confidence, *joie de vivre*, need for recognition, even 'heartiness' and trust, however.) Just so there should be no confusion between the heart organ (small 'h') and the Heart energy or Heart meridian (capital 'H'). An underfunctioning Heart meridian does not necessarily mean that the heart is in a dangerous condition.

(Speaking of the organs, it must be remembered that the basic Western functions of the organs — for example the kidneys, in formation of urine — have not been elaborated in Chinese medicine. Instead, Chinese medicine deals with energetic function and is less concerned with organic pathology. This will become clearer later. Consequently, traditional Chinese medicine can take longer, and may outwardly seem less effective, than Western treatment in *acute* organic pathological conditions. That said, it is surprising how many apparently urgent operations have been averted by means of the right oriental 'energetic thrust', the patients being returned to live comfortably with themselves. However, there are no easy answers, and there can be bad practitioners of acupuncture and good and humane 'Western' doctors. There are 'bad' astrologers too. Unfortunately, as always, many letters after a name do not guarantee a wise head!)

Here are two ancient systems of thought. Both synthesize; both look for underlying patterns that predispose to suffering; both point to strengths and weaknesses in body and mind — and perhaps spirit too; and both are intimately connected with the changing flux of the seasons and cycles of energy in life. Astrology should find in Chinese medicine a better vehicle for medical understanding than in its Western counterpart. Perhaps an appreciation of the combined strengths will bring closer the day when Western medical training embraces them, and is thereby enriched.

The Cycle of Phases

If disease is the inability to change, or a blockage in the body's adaptability to new conditions, one way to consider health is in the form of a cycle, any phase of which is the result of the previous phase and the source of the next. Ill health arises when we cannot proceed out of one phase.

What have become known as the Five Elements are here described as the Five Phases, not only to distinguish the Chinese term from the astrological term 'Elements' but also because it is a more accurate description. The astrological Elements, Fire, Earth, Air and Water are four separate states, each with its own strengths and weaknesses, and each Element is subdivided into three parts (cardinal, fixed, mutable) which describe modes of action. But Fire does not turn into Water, or Air or Earth, because they are separate polarities or situations.

In the cycle of phases, each phase has associations, but there are moving and changing and controlling aspects, and ill health occurs when 'stuck' in a phase.

Although there are five phases (Fire, Earth, Metal, Water and Wood), it is easier to understand their action by first taking Fire, Metal, Water and Wood, and astrologers must resist the temptation to regard these as corresponding to the Elements in Western astrology, equating Fire with *Fire*, and Water with *Water*, and fitting *Earth* and *Air* into Metal and Wood. Such attempts will only frustrate deeper understanding.

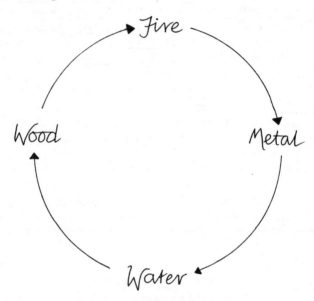

Diagram 1. 4 Phase Diagram.

Wood

Wood describes the quickening period of the year, day or life; we have expectations and plans to look forward to. We arise in the morning, rested after our sleep, full of energy for the day ahead, minds buzzing with things to do, and if we regulate ourselves correctly we attend to our gastro-intestinal system and then, suitably fuelled, we can move ahead.

In the course of the year, spring brings green sprouts, wind, warmth and movement. The buds, dormant throughout winter, now expand and seeds push upwards towards the light.

So in terms of energy, Wood is light, moving, expanding to explore its surroundings. Its strength comes from its adaptability and ability to organize itself and its environment. It is an exciting phase, full of tension which, if cleared smoothly, gives a hopeful outlook and a cheerful opportunism.

Fire
But Wood burns. Or, better put, spring gives way to summer, the eager anticipation of youth to maturity. After the morning comes noon, the height of the sun's power. Here there is the warmth towards which Wood pushed, the laughter of friendship and love (not just the obsession of 'falling in love') and the flowers — the descendants of the buds. Here we enjoy ourselves, and in liking ourselves, glorying in our splendour, we can like and give love to others, and in so doing become one with them. Our radiant energy flows outwards, and in others is reflected back to us, and we see the true life within us. This is the phase when what we planned comes to fruition, and we see that our creation is good. It is a time of integration and wholeness, all parts functioning together — spirit, mind and body working together and at peace. So the burning of Wood gives a steady warm glow.

Metal
After the glowing embers, the ashes, those fond remembrances of the evening and twilight, when we look back on the day, and we sort through memories of our actions, learning from our experiences and discarding what is no longer needed. We clear up the mess we have made from living, we wash and clear the tables and we settle down to do chores and to make space for ourselves. The flowers have produced their fruit which we harvest, and the stalks need to be pruned, ploughed, composted or burned, and the grain stored. We need to dredge the lakes, clear the drains and gutters and put the garbage where it can be used. Rubbish is only useless when it is in the wrong place: the earth has a use for it, though it may take time. Those useless stalks make good compost, and faeces make excellent manure for the future.

In this phase we see our children mature, and we hand over our activities to them, retiring to enjoy our savings, whether spiritual or material. Now we can look back with wisdom and, given a receptive audience, teach from the strength of our experience, and help those who need it, tempering with justice the over-enthusiasm and indulgences of those younger. This is a very ordinary phase when all things have reached resolution, are in their place, and life continues in tranquillity.

Take the meaning of Metal as being the minerals and values that return to the earth to give it quality.

Water

After the twilight, night; time to rest or, in winter, to hibernate. A time of waiting. Nothing much happens; we try to keep warm, but things slow and ice up. Seeds, planted at the end of the year, just wait. The land lies fallow. But in winter there is a great energy of water and cold wind, but the nights are longer and we see less of them. If exposed to them, we die, and we die when we have exhausted the energy of our span of life. But whereas the other phases express kinetic energies, here all is potential: 'God moving over the face of the water'. The period of pre-life and post-life, a time of dreamless sleep, recovering energy. Here we must not be impatient, we must not force new growth, or we risk harming the growing foetus, turning it out before it is ready. The seeds of experience sink into our minds and are integrated into new forms of possibility. Only the morrow, the next spring or the new life will show how things turn out, but here all is promise. The minerals and compost and manure have returned to the earth to enrich it, but the earth takes time to absorb them, and while it does so all is still, no life shows.

The new Cycle

And then the cycle repeats itself. The wind's nature changes and the buds return, the waiting broods no more. Nature takes another breath.

But there is more in the diagram. Fire and Water form a polarity, as do Wood and Metal, and each end of the polarity balances its opposite. If the Water phase lacked time to recover, then the Fire will not burn so steadily, as some of its energy will be needed to compensate, as a plant forced to produce flowers throughout the winter cannot also be expected to live out its full span. And if the Fire burns too brightly, the mind cannot settle in sleep. The adaptability and mutability of Wood needs the experience and strength of Metal behind it or it may exhaust itself in crazy experiments; whilst Metal needs the enthusiasm and ambition of Wood to prevent it from falling into melancholy and obsessions with the past. Very often in illness, if one phase is upset, the opposite phase also becomes unbalanced, and intermediate phases strive to appear normal.

The diagram also shows the sorts of disease we are prone to. Young people are on the left side of the cycle, and their problems are nearly always those of over-function, over-reaction, growing too fast, accident from lack of experience, fever (Fire, burning too brightly) or early disease so exhausting that they take much longer to recover, or are left with its after-effects for ever. Thus severely exhausting disease in early childhood may cripple a particular phase such as Water/Fire — for many years.

At the opposite end of life, the problem of depression, (which it should be said can arise from imbalance at any phase), is usually manifest on the Wood-Metal polarity. Depression signifies energy that is held back and does not flow freely. In someone young, or with good life energy, the chances are that this is only a passing problem, even if acute; at any rate there is plenty to look forward to, and if the right key to unlock the energy can be found, there is every chance of a return to a healthy zest for life. But in someone old, in the Metal-Water phase of the cycle, the life energy is declining and memories, not hopes, form the main area of thought. Depression, like grief, is often due to unexpressed anger, but whether true or not, the effect is one of frustration, with the Wood energy tightening up and Metal unable to budge. So prospects for cure are less hopeful, especially where an outlet (Wood) for creativity such as work has dried up, and the individual has never been able to develop a sense of self-worth (Metal) — indeed may have been running away from confronting his feelings about himself all his life. Here Metal never developed, leaving Wood to compensate. When Wood's outlets disappeared, Metal has no strength to carry forward the life. (See Chart I.)

Case 1: Male, 73
All the personal planets save ☽ are on the ascending half of his chart. A teacher and organizer of teachers, this patient had his whole interest in life terminated when he retired. Most Sagittarians have many interests and a willingness to learn, but ♃ lacks vibrant aspects save to Medium Coeli and Ascendant. Without a useful career here, it runs out of steam, and the heavy weight of ♄♃ and ☉♏ begin to manifest. Saturn is T-square ♅ and ♆ giving it additional lethargy, so that perhaps we should say that the ground which this man has made for himself enforces restriction; his disciplined habits of a lifetime now fence him in. Additionally, ♄ is alone in its quarter of the horoscope, giving it, at its time of life, greater authority unless balanced by other factors. But save the T-square, ♄ has no other strong aspects.

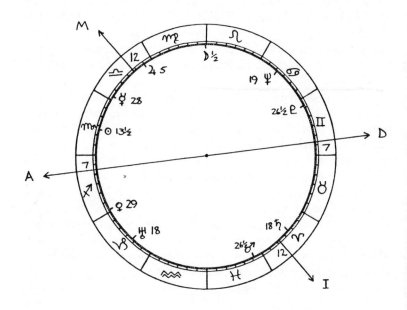

Chart 1. Male, 73.

Both ♀ and ♂, which give the value of relationships and the force of vibrancy, are in T-square with ♇, deepening their energies and making them less able to be directed extrovertly. The aspect ♀★☿ would have been important in early life and shows, together with ☽□A, how important is the woman in this man's life, as a source of inspiration. But in psychological terms we have to doubt whether he will have put down an effective personality base for himself for his old age, when he is likely to become depressed.

In terms of his energy, if for the moment we say that ♄ has to do with his sense of belonging in a secure environment — in this case his body — then he is going to find that environment a depressing place, one that is unreliable and somewhat uncomfortable to live out his days in. At the other end of the chart, almost unaspected ♃ will help to pick him up for brief periods of respite during which he is likely to become over optimistic. But as ♄ is not properly integrated into the rest of the personality, they are unlikely to last.

Depression, however, though present, was not his presenting complaint, which was a strange sensation of wetness on the soles of his feet when standing with socks and shoes on. Western medicine had no diagnosis save a vague form of 'peripheral neuritis'. In traditional Chinese medicine the palms of the hands and the soles of the feet are related to the liver energy, and this chart shows someone whose mind became obsessively hypochondriacal over a foot sensation associated with an almost unaspected ♃, whose body, ♄, lacked ability to learn new ways. It got stuck in the past, which we might here equate with the 4th house.

This man discovered for himself that the only thing that worked was change: whenever he encountered a new treatment the energy, if it worked at all, did so for only a few weeks. This points to ☽ and ☿, the two planets that were 'well' aspected, both of which are moving and mutable, and parting from aspect with ♇, the only heavy planet either aspects.

In this case prognosis was poor, as once ♄ — the body — had fixed itself a pattern, it would be hard to change.

Earth

Four phases have been described, yet none could exist without Earth,

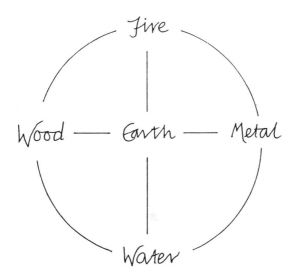

Diagram 2. 4 Phases with Earth.

the place where life exists. It can therefore be placed at the centre of the circle, as each part of the cycle interacts with it. From one point of view, the cycle shows four aspects of Earth, so Earth *is* in the cycle.

Before going on to describe it, it must be said that there are two paradigms. If Earth is taken as in Diagram 2, then whenever any phase is upset, it can be supported from Earth, its foundation.
But if it is taken as part of the five-phase diagram (Diagram 3) it is usually placed after Fire and before Metal, although there are arguments for placing it elsewhere in the cycle.

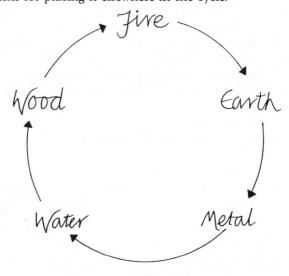

Diagram 3. 5 Phase Diagram.

Consider it at first at the centre. Here it forms a polarity with each one of the four phases, so that any of them can injure Earth, and vice versa: that is to say that Earth either gets unbalanced in sympathy, or the cause of its imbalance is directly attributable to one of the other phases. Here, 'Earth' refers mainly to the organs and associations of Earth, rather than the Earth meridians.
In the five-phase cycle, the Earth phase follows usually after Fire on the grounds, amongst others, that it represents the fruits and grains of the harvest time or late summer, the maturing period, parenthood (nurturing and *protecting* period, we should say). It does not seem to have such a clear-cut time of day, and the fact that some diagrams place it for instance between Water and Wood, instead of

between Fire and Earth, shows that it can also be seen as the time between rising in the morning and setting off for work, when we feed and attend to the calls of nature.

Problems

What then are the problems each phase suffers?

Wood phase imbalance

Imagine yourself in a car, driving from home to work in the morning. You have listed certain things you must do as regards home — such as buy food, or ring up about a repair — but mainly you are thinking of the coming meetings, decisions and events, of how you will deal with them and for what contingencies you must prepare. This may be particularly relevant on a Monday, or after a holiday. Now suppose that an accident causes a traffic jam, and you grind to a halt. If there is an important early meeting which you must attend, you will grow tense. (The fact that you may have methods of alleviating tension and of relaxing is irrelevant.) This tension, due to frustration of your forward motion, is the body's response, and the four-phase diagram shows that it is healthy. You may become irritable, especially if someone hoots their horn at you. Usually you will find that muscles are tensing, particularly in the upper part of the body; shoulders hunch, jaws and neck muscles tighten. Like a bean sprout watered, warmed and well lit, but constrained behind glass, your body pushes its energy upwards, and you may get a headache, or sore eyes, especially if long delayed.

When traffic starts again, these responses subside and you may even be able to laugh at yourself — the appropriate outlet in terms of the phases, as Fire (laughter) follows Wood (tension).

But suppose now that your future depended on the decision of another, who refused to commit himself, and that you were unable to make any move in your life until he took the necessary action; or that the action of a colleague always made you tense, or that the amount of work to be done always exceeded your capabilities and that new requirements were always being made of you unexpectedly. You would have to get used to living in a state of tension. Your mind might be razor sharp, but you would find it hard to relax, and could expect sleep and eating habits to suffer — the latter because regular food intake was disturbed, the former because your mind would always be teeming with new possibilities and contingency plans. Your position might make it impossible for you to vent your frustration save in sport, and you might well find that spasms and cramps upset your ability to exercise freely and easily.

Internal causes of Wood imbalance

The above describes what begins to happen when mind or emotion is upset, and cannot realign itself. The body has become trapped in a particular kind of tension, where there are spasms and contractions, and energy is felt as pain that is acutely uncomfortable, rising up towards the head. The internal cause of the imbalance is here 'Anger', although it should be noted that 'frustration' and other descriptions such as 'uncertainty' or 'being neutralized' are just as useful. Equally, some patients suffering from these same terrible and griping pains (often of a distending nature, particularly if abdominal) appear to be the very opposite of angry: indeed they never stop smiling, or being nice. These patients cannot express their 'anger', though their bodies do.

If the above is caused by an internal cause, what happens when the cause is external? Here is a Chinese term that covers a very wide range of experiences, and is often the first cause of externally created disease: *Wind*.

The wind blows: it sends us good and bad weather, hot and cold, dry and damp, strong gales and soft breezes. It describes moving air, and it is predominantly this aspect of changeability that is dangerous, for it is sudden changes in the weather that bring ill health, such as moving say from hot to cold environments without having the strength to combat their effects.

The wind also brings bacteria and viruses, which the Chinese could not see but called 'invisible worms'.

Modern air-conditioning is a boon, but it throws all sorts of small currents of air around us which, given an appropriate gap in the defences, will enter and give us their characteristic symptoms. In Hong Kong, where some of the old beliefs remain, many Chinese women refuse to give birth to their babies in hospital wards where there is air-conditioning, so strong is their fear of 'Wind'. With modern techniques this is probably carrying things too far, although it illustrates the close relationship between 'Wind' ('Wood') and 'fear' of 'Water' association. (No doubt also, a modern, Western hospital is full of terrors for a Chinese woman parted from her domestic way of life, though rapid rises in living standards in Hong Kong are probably counteracting these old beliefs now.)

We reject such superstitions too easily nowadays: they are founded on experience, no matter that they have been taken to ridiculous lengths. We, perhaps, go too far in the opposite direction; with technological advances we believe we control our environment, but if we think we can control our bodies, we fool ourselves. As the drug companies know well, their drugs wear out in effectiveness, needing more powerful replacements, which if they are not curative, become palliative and later reach the stage where we are physically or psychologically dependent upon them. Are we then controlling them, or they us?

Symptoms of external Wind
The beginnings of a cold or influenza have Wind symptoms which move, change, run around all over the body. So there is for example sneezing, shivering, hot and cold feelings up and down the back, pains that move around, now in the cheek, then in the forehead, then elbow. There is often a dislike of wind and intolerance of draughts. Usually the upper half of the body is affected, and there may be spontaneous perspiration, a headache, nasal obstruction and a sore, dry or itchy throat.

Because Wind moves, its signature in the body is one of movement, so look for spasmodic motions, twitches and rigidities (e.g. of stiff neck), tremors and twisted facial muscles, grimacings, facial or eye tics, and deviation of the eyes.

In practice, Wind often occurs with other external factors such as 'cold', 'damp', 'phlegm', 'dryness' and 'heat'.

The cause of this is, traditionally, exposure to wind or draughts, especially if the body is cooling from a heated state, for example if there has been sweating. Here the pores of the skin (associated with Metal) are open to invasion of wind. Wood and Metal form a polarity so 'Wood overcomes Metal' one could say.

In astrological terminology, we expect aspects mainly from progressed ☽, transiting ♃ or ♅, each of which betokens change when signs of external Wind manifest.

Fire phase imbalance
A man who feels he is healthy and in command of his faculties and life, who is beginning to enjoy the successful outcome of his plans and efforts, should be happy and enviable. But suppose he receives bad news; the death of a spouse or the collapse of an important investment; or he has an accident that floors him. Suddenly he can no longer depend on what he was sure of, and there is a gap in his life; his self-confidence is shaken. No longer can he be the magnanimous, big-hearted man he thought himself; his control slips.

Imagine, next, someone unable to make satisfactory relationships because he cannot appear confident of himself. That shield of warm companionability and co-operation that we need to operate in a civilized society is lacking, and he shrinks from giving too much of himself for fear of losing all.

Consider another type: smart, strong-willed and well-groomed; exuding self-confidence, he strives mightily at whatever he does and avoids physical work; he is mentally strong — but there is an underlying nervousness about himself, and a tendency to be over-sensitive. When things go wrong, this sensitivity and nervousness turn into hysteria and paranoia as he loses control, even if outwardly remaining icily calm. But inside, as he telephones his doctor for a 'check-up', he is panicking; and as he arranges a time, he is pouring with sweat. At a later stage, he no longer makes any attempt to seem calm and confident, but retreats into a shell of insecurity, where a constant refrain is often 'What is happening to me?' and a feeling of having been let down by friends. One of the reasons he feels like this is that he has tried to manage too many things for too long, his pride preventing him from admitting any kind of weakness or inability to cope. Also he makes promises too easily, and cannot keep all of them.

Here the big-heartedness goes too far, and the Fire exhausts itself or burns unevenly. In other words, it cannot provide that maturity that gives balance and control. Worry and continual concern over his affairs and relationships upsets the harmony of his life, and he goes to pieces.

Symptoms of internal Fire imbalance

Emotional distress; worry, nervousness, fidgetiness, restlessness, mental confusion, even inability to speak, with underlying fear and anxiety, form the mental background. (Traditional Chinese medicine is actually far more precise than this, but a broad picture is all that is necessary here.)

On the physical level, common complaints are an unsteady, intermittent pulse, or palpitations. If the condition is one of qi or yang deficiency (see Chapter 7) then there is low energy, shallow breathing or shortness of breath and pallor, and probably chills and cold limbs and feet. There may be profuse sweating, especially during the day.

If the condition is yin deficient, then night sweats predominate and there may be dizziness and a feeling of heat in the afternoon, and insomnia or sleep much disturbed by dreams and worries. Getting off to sleep is a problem in both types (they daren't 'let go').

In strong people the face goes red, and there is soreness and swelling or ulceration of teeth and gums, with painful burning urine. Here there is delirium and nightmare and a feverish sensation. There may be trembling.

Symptoms of external Fire imbalance 'Heat'

More common in hot climates, although being brought home more often by holiday-makers lacking awareness or respect for local health customs in hot countries, external Fire imbalance problems do occur in northern and cold countries, and are normally due to exposure to heat (e.g. the sun, a hot radiator, sauna, hot sand or rocks) when tired, (although there is also another cause arising from cold and dampness). There is fever, and the body feels lethargic, heavy and painful. Usually limbs feel icy cold, there is a dry mouth and an awful headache, frequently throbbing, with depression and nausea.

Another kind of problem arises from heat, which produces thick, hot smelly (foul) excretions. Diarrhoea is urgent and the anus burns. Stools are very smelly and any mucus is often thick and yellow. The pulse is fast.

The imagery of 'Heat' and 'Fire' helps us to understand the next stage, where heat 'dries' — leading to dry mouth and dry stools (with painful bowel movements and tearing sensations in the anus on passing) and thirst.

Heat also stirs up the 'wind' and disturbs fluids, just as the afternoon on-land breeze in tropical climates can be very strong, whipping up quite large waves. Here there is high fever, delirium, convulsions and stiffness in the upper body. Any virus or germ like scarlet fever thrives in these conditions if it can find them, but the condition can exist without the germ, and the germ can also help produce the symptoms. Whipping up the fluids here refers to the 'Blood', specifically Liver Blood, leading to haemorrhage, for example nose bleeds, skin eruptions and rashes.

'Fire' is a more severe form of 'Heat'. In a person able to produce such symptoms, we would find a fever without a chill, and the patient would be red-faced, with probably red sclera, urine and tongue. There might be hot, burning skin infections or ulcerations.

Symptoms of internal Fire imbalance are problems of shen (spirit) in the mental sphere; where exernal Fire disturbs the shen, we get mania and delirium.

Broadly speaking, then, external 'Heat' affects the throat, lungs, gastrointestinal tract and skin, then the urine, sclera and blood circulation, and only then the mind and emotions, whereas internal

'Heat' starts from the emotions and moves into the body via the circulation, eventually affecting the skin and the gastrointestinal system.

Further considerations

Strictly speaking, under this heading should also be mentioned the difference between 'Full' Heat and 'Empty' Heat. In general, 'Empty' Heat is associated with an internal condition known as 'deficiency of yin' whereas 'Full' Heat derives from external factors. Examples of predominantly deficiency of yin (= 'Empty' Heat) situations are diabetes and lung tuberculosis, whereas 'Full' Heat situations are those of fever and delirium caused from the outside. The distinction should be clearer after reading Chapter 7, on yin and yang.

Metal phase imbalance

If a healthy person reaps what he needs and disposes of the rest, then an unhealthy person takes — or values — the wrong things, and saddles himself with trash, which he cannot or will not get rid of.

Trash, like beauty, depends on the beholder. A dung heap is a wonderful, creative, not to say satisfying place, if you happen to be a dung fly. Much current psychological thinking would have us believe that the rubbish we carry about in ourselves and conceal from others — whether it be grim memories or constipated faeces — gives us experience through which we can grow. Traditional Chinese medicine agrees, but puts it another way: by giving up that rubbish we enrich our environment and make space for ourselves to grow within, and for our environment to move on outside. So, by withholding, we poison our lives and impoverish the lives of those around us. We give ourselves no room to take in the new, and we deprive the world of our own experience.

We 'play God' (or God 'plays us') when we give out and take in without hindrance, but when we cling to what we have and refuse to share, we are of no value to ourselves or to others.

So Metal is about making a space; and curiously, the freer that space the more we trust and value ourselves. The more we cling on to what that space contains, the more blocked and despicable we feel. A metal is of no intrinsic value until someone wants it and uses it; then it can give strength.

Consider some examples of people who are blocked up. As we grow older, we have more memories, and our ability to pick and choose them diminishes. Some people, even though young, are so blocked that they can discuss nothing but themselves. It is not that

Go THRU IT, NOT JUST To IT —

you HAVE no feelings

they are selfishly self-seeking, but that their problems form too large an obstacle for them to see or pass beyond. In the old, memories often form an increasing part of their life, and if we bemoan passed times we cling to them. Those who have been brought up to believe that it is bad form to cry, to caress, to admit grief or sorrow or anger or laughter or fear or the need for sympathy (or even some of these) will find life stilted and grey. They will feel life passing them by, and they will grieve. And they will be right. Life *is* passing them by, because they won't let it pass through them — where it may hurt a bit.

The English 'stiff upper lip' is always mentioned here, and in its place it has value. That determination to maintain dignity and standards won many adherents and much respect around the world, even if it is now fashionable to decry it. No doubt in its place it was valuable — it *did* impress — but the mistake which we impute to it (whether rightly or wrongly is not here the issue) was that it was carried over into life as a standard that all English men — and many of their women — should hold before them as an example of how life should be lived. So nobody was allowed to show his or her feelings and, being prevented from sharing them, got stuck with them, stopping any more mature feelings from growing. Hence the immature emotional life and experience of many who have been forced into such a 'military' discipline. No wonder they were left with such an infantile emotional facility.

Another aspect of this is that it is quite hard work carrying all this unreleased energy through life. So people who are downhearted and depressed about themselves often feel lacking in energy, which reflects in their attitudes and hopes of betterment. Frequently they get angry and bitter at their lot — which can actually be a sign of improvement — for they might do something about it!

So the Metal phase is frequently not functioning properly if we are stuck with debris that we do not want; even more so if we are not aware of it. Phlegm and mucus and intestines that cannot expel their contents come at least partly under this, as do lumps under the skin. The organs of excretion, skin, lungs, bladder and large intestine are all potentially affected. (However, it should be noted that phlegm and mucus are not, strictly speaking, manufactured by a faulty Metal energy; but they may be stored by it.)

Nearly all Metal types are searching for something better, and they have a great appetite for new and unusual ideas and philosophies. This search is an attempt to compensate for their own sense of unworthiness, their lack of quality and value. Unfortunately they are not very good at dumping old ideas, so they often end up with a crazy collection of muddled theories.

Their problem is that they want to be a part of everything and to be loved and loveable, but they don't feel worthy. So they keep looking for ways to improve themselves.

Before discussing some of the symptoms of internal Metal imbalance, let us consider how a well-functioning Metal phase enriches our lives. We feel clean and open to new experiences; we can accept what life gives us, because we are happy with ourselves. We are not rubbish. We have a right to be here and we look forward to receiving new ideas, concepts and friends, not to mention air, the *Qigong* breath of life itself, because we know we have room and need for it, and because we know that we can dump what we do not need without rancour. The skin, our outer line of defence, and our lungs, the first major inner organ to receive, come under Metal. Clear skin and a well-modulated, powerful voice, are signs of healthy qi, especially Lung qi. To breathe properly, we must stand upright and look life in the face. If we stand round-shouldered, we cannot breathe easily, and we tighten ourselves round our memories, rather than being, like a laughing child, open to whatever may come. If our Metal qi works well, our system functions easily and naturally.

Symptoms of internal Metal imbalance

Usually there is slowness, due to inability to react to stimuli automatically. More important, there is tiredness, obstinacy, depression and a dislike of talking, a feeling of unworthiness and a tendency to avoid society. The cause is often a long-standing worry or grief. The patient frequently catches colds and suffers many respiratory complaints. The face is white, the skin is dry, and he feels cold. The voice is weak, and he is short of breath. This is a picture of deficient Metal qi, and is due to internal causes unless Metal has been weakened by repeated external evils over a long time, for example tuberculosis. (But in this case yin would be weakened also, giving a kind of weak, fiery nature which exhausts itself easily but gets wonderful and original ideas. It feels warmer in the afternoon when cheeks may flush and there may be thirst or a dry mouth. These types are usually thin-bodied.)

Symptoms of external Metal imbalance

The Metal phase governs a number of different areas; the respiratory system (including lung, trachea, bronchi, throat and nose) the large intestine — important for absorption of water and elimination of waste — and the skin, a barrier but also a means of breathing and elimination.

Where 'Metal' is imbalanced by external causes, the energies of these organs are disturbed and syndromes such as 'Invasion of lung by pathogenic Wind' arise, an occurrence familiar to all who have suffered a 'cold'. This is more fully discussed in Chapter 4.

Water phase imbalance

Imagine yourself tired, but unable to rest or sleep. Imagine that just as you are turning out your bedside light, the telephone rings and you have to return to work instead of sleeping. Imagine that you have completed a tiring mental task but that instead of rest, you must begin another. Imagine your sleep patterns continually upset by the demands of sleepless children, or worrying business problems or some other form of inquisition. Visualize the effect on your body of prolonged use of pep-pills, of stimulants such as coffee, to keep you awake and alert.

After a period of sleep deprivation, we become less sure of ourselves and of our ability to make considered moves. For a while our nerves are overexcitable and oversensitive. Our minds become overactive. We become irritable, our hearing more acute. We may find that our hands tremble and our faces twitch. Probably we become more hungry, and we eat and drink too fast. Heartbeat becomes irregular, or palpitates nervously from even a small stimulus. We find our minds go blank suddenly, or that we have done something we do not remember doing. We tire quickly.

And when we are allowed to sleep naturally? The sleep will be restless; fitful images will prevent us from slipping into calm untroubled slumber. Only when we have rested for a while or been on holiday will our ability to sleep deeply return.

The state of vacancy, or we might even call it vacuity, has a place in creation. We need to be able to enter that state easily. Who knows what happens there? Wherever 'I' am, I am not present in my body. You cannot learn much about my personality when I am fast asleep. But this state of unconsciousness is the closest we get to the state of death. We may infer that this nightly surrender to the state closest to pure yin, a state of mere physical presence, a state uniquely shared with every living creature, somehow reconnects us with our lifespring itself. We awake refreshed, ready to learn and experience anew.

Earth phase imbalance

The Earth orb of energy encompasses almost anything to do with nutrition. It includes the gastrointestinal tract from mouth to anus, the whole process of digestion, the area of the body from base of sternum to umbilicus including stomach, spleen, pancreas, duodenum, jejunum, ileum, gall bladder and liver, though Wood phase is also involved with gall bladder and liver. It includes the umbilical cord and the nutrients in a pregnant mother's uterus, her breasts and her protective motherliness.

We all know the nurturing sorts of person: they have a sympathetic ear and a caring attitude. Doctors, nurses, teachers, politicians and acupuncturists, for example, who lose this side of themselves soon lose their customers. There are many who see their life's work in this field: it is a big one. Farmers, bankers, office workers, those who nurse and heal, teachers especially of those who have not yet reached puberty, cooks, the whole food and clothing retail market, librarians, herbalists and chemists, to suggest but a few; also those involved in energy transportation and news or information dissemination. In short, those who supply our everyday needs and keep us going, yet who work mainly behind the scenes, their services largely unrecognized save by the everyday needs we place upon them; the whole of the service industry.

They are our backbone and support; often their jobs are dull and repetitive, but without them we should have no reserves and no civilization. They are mankind about its daily business of keeping the human race going and procreating.

Babies emerge from the womb needing to survive — which means eliciting food, warmth and tender loving care from their parents. There is no shortage of individuals who never had enough of this in childhood — or behave as if they didn't — who as adults go on clamouring for this attention: and all the more so if sick. So to take just a few examples, anyone over-concerned — for whatever reason — with anything to do with their nutrition is potentially imbalanced in Earth: those who are too fat, too thin, overeat or undereat, and those whose gastro-intestinal tract causes them pain and discomfort, and who not infrequently believe certain foods are good or bad.

Just as much involved are those who feel out of touch with reality, who think too much and worry endlessly about their life and their state of health. Even exercise and keep-fit fanatics are included!

Earth reaches everywhere, partly through its process of nutrition and protection. It is also the carrier of energy. It is transformation and transportation and, after taking food to all parts, removes the trash. So build-up of unwanted matter, whether in the form of surplus fat, or oedema, bruised tissue that has swollen, lymph-glands that are choked or enlarged, varicose veins, phlegm stuck in the nose and fluid in the knee — all may be due to an inactive Earth energy. On the emotional front, there is a kind of heavy, turgid depression, self-blaming, apt to wallow in misery and unable to see a way out; often tearful, it looks for security and sympathy, and is peevish, irritable, jealous and touchy. These people brood over trivia. They feel dull and lethargic, and frequently have all sorts of fears and anxieties. They often have poor circulation, and their tissues and muscles are relaxed or weak. They lack stamina and easily strain tendons. Altogether there is a feeling of congestion.

There are so many individual varieties of discomfort under Earth that one can give only a few indications of the personality types. But underlying them all, on both physical and mental levels, are the ideas firstly of digestion, with all its connotations of nutrition, and secondly that of movement (= transportation) meaning direction of body fluids and energy through the body, including removal of waste materials. (Body fluids here include, amongst others, blood — arterial and venous — lymph fluids, hormones, water, sweat, tears, and absorption and exudations of mucous membranes.)

Symptoms of internal Earth imbalance

Where there is a deficiency of Earth qi there is melancholy, mental fatigue, lassitude, obsession — often with the past, or with the state of health, or with details. There is general dissatisfaction, poor memory, sleepiness (yet sleep is poor), and either a lack of appetite for life in general as well as for food, or a tendency to eat too much and too fast, and to work whilst doing so. The brain is always going, chuntering on about work or the state of health. Worriers, who enjoy having something to worry about. Their problems arise over a long period of overeating, or irregular eating — meaning meals at irregular times, or taken in a hurry, or snacks taken at odd moments followed by enormous meals which the body neither needs nor can cope with — such as late at night. The food itself may be of poor quality or not fresh. (An additional factor nowadays may be chemicals added to foods to preserve or enhance their flavours. Artificial colouring agents sometimes lead to hyperactivity, for example.) Similarly, excessive or voracious eating in particular harms the Earth energy. By excessive is meant eating more than is needed for the lifestyle and energetic output. So big eaters need plenty of exercise! Irregular food intake also means eating food that is too hot or too cold. A surprising number of gynaecological problems are accentuated by eating too much chilled food, or fresh cold salads. But drinking iced fruit juice when one is overheated — say from heavy exercise in summer heat — can also damage Earth energy. These latter causes are external factors, but if indulged in regularly produce the same situation — a deficiency of Earth qi (= in this case, Spleen qi).

The other main cause of Earth phase problems is overwork, either physical or mental. The former cause is less common in the West than the latter, but physical over-exertion certainly exists, and occurs most frequently when food is eaten immediately before heavy exertion, with no intermediate rest. It also occurs when taking too much exercise before warming up: here one could say that we overstrain our muscles (Earth) before we have warmed up (Fire). Exercise enthusiasts take note! More important, however, is excessive thinking; 'Overwork injures the Spleen'. Amongst its other duties, the Spleen rules concentration, memory and cogitation, the abilities to reflect and to distinguish.

On the whole, a long period of excessive work or mental strain is required to harm Earth.

Protracted chronic disease also damages Spleen qi. Physically, weak Spleen qi means hypofunction of the spleen in its process of transforming and transporting, and weakness of its related tissues and organs. Symptoms include a sallow complexion (sometimes yellow), anorexia, abdominal distension, loose stools, oedema and, of course, general lassitude. The oedema occurs in arms and legs usually. Clearly, weak Spleen qi mainly affects the function of the intestines in absorbing and distributing food, leading by failure to increased fluid in the intestines, consequently anorexia, abdominal distension and loose stools.

'Weakness of Spleen produces damp; excess damp leads to loose stools.' Here in particular it is the transportation of water that goes awry. But weakness in transportation leads to deficient fluids and energy reaching the extremities, causing by their absence weakness, heaviness and lassitude in the limbs. Long continued, this leads to emaciation of the arms and legs, and sometimes a bloated or enlarged abdomen, frequently found in old people who have harmed their Earth energy over too long a period. Sallowness, sometimes with other signs of anaemia, also comes from weak Earth transforming power, as the blood is not properly nourished.

A more thorough examination of this and other energies is undertaken in later chapters. The point to remember with the Earth energy is that we are apt to overlook its importance, just because it is such an automatic fact of life. With Wood energy we expand and develop; in Fire we grow to maturity and enjoy ourselves; in Metal we look for quality and value; in Water we find will-power and potential. But in Earth we vegetate and turn food into energy, we think and reflect; hence the importance of relaxed meditation, carefree trust, calm, unworried and unhurried behaviour if we get ill — for only then will our Earth energy be able to exert its calming influence and form an integrated base from which other energies can flow.

Summary of the Phases

Water: We derive our lifespring, our energy and will for life. We start from pure potential. When in sleep we dream, but do not accomplish in reality. We begin here from a position of minimum activity but maximum possibility, so this can be seen as the period of winter, of sleep, or pre-birth and very early childhood.

Wood: Like a released spring our energy for growth and development and learning resounds in us. We are full of plans. We want to explore, to expand our experience, to act, to move, to thrust, to sever. This is spring, morning, puberty, our twenties and thirties.

Fire: Enjoyment, laughter; no longer the mad rush of ideas, the urgent need to prove ourselves, but the pleasure of loving, living and creating. Summer, midday and the period when we begin to receive appreciation from our peers.

Metal: Pleasures are now part of us. We have refined the will, the urge and the joy into our quality of life. The value people place on us, our sterling virtues, our resilience and openness to new ideas, tempered with wisdom, integrate to give us empathy, yet strength to avoid being overpowered, and a sense of uniqueness and our rightful place in the world. The period is autumn, the end of the day, the time in life where we reflect on our past and on our needs for the present and the future, whether they may be in the form of investments, friends or lovely surroundings and possessions. This is the period before night, and rest, and a new beginning.

Earth: Underlying all the other energies is the vehicle we live in. It gives us a place to live, a home to rest in, a ground on which to stand, and memories on which to draw. In a general sense it is our means of being present, so it is not only our home and our backbone, but our form of communication with the rest of humanity. Our body combines with all other humans to form races and nationalities. Is it any wonder that nationality, boundaries and food, agriculture, possessions, health and education have always been such emotive issues? But in themselves they are not emotive; they are just there, and without them we should not exist. But they form the ever-present exigencies of life: we may ignore our bodies, but we fight for the right to live in them!

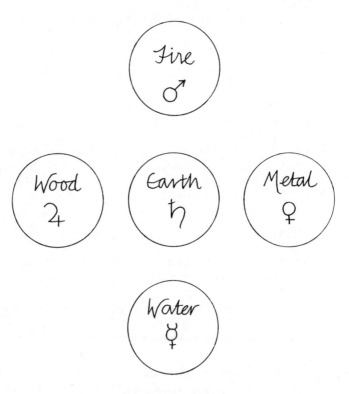

Diagram 4. Astrological Correlations

Astrological Significations

The Chinese have handed down certain planetary associations with the phases:

Water	☿	Mercury
Wood	♃	Jupiter
Fire	♂	Mars
Metal	♀	Venus
Earth	♄	Saturn

Some of these associations are obvious to an astrologer, in particular ♃ with Wood. The least obvious are Water, and ☿, Metal and ♀, indeed some would say these correspondences should be reversed but, as it is hoped the following will show, the Chinese made the right connections, at least from their point of view. (Some astrologers may have to make some adjustments in their understanding of the planets!)

The question of Sun ☉, Moon ☽, Uranus ♅, Neptune ♆ and Pluto ♇ is discussed later.

2.

JUPITER ♃

Jupiter in a chart represents an ability to grow in physique and understanding. It has to do with our ability to visualize and to imagine, to hope and to have faith; future orientated, it carries risk. It governs expansion through growth, exploration and an urge towards something larger than ourselves, whether it be a group or a fortune. It has much to do with the spatial right side of our brains. It represents our capacity to learn how to compensate for inadequacies, to improve ourselves, to go beyond the humdrum everyday routine of life, to create movement and excitement and visions of vistas new.

To the extent that our lives proceed forward amicably and optimistically we offend no sense of justice. But when we are presented — either by our own excess, exaggeration, conceit, procrastination and even lawlessness, or by external force whose might exceeds our own — then we have to change and develop if we wish to succeed. Seen in this light, traditional rulership over justice, mercy, morals and a sense of law and order, is not the stultifying bureaucratic law of red tape, but that of an active sense of fair play for all, and a religious conviction of faith and hope in a better-ordered world. Taken to excess — a highly Jovian word and, it may be said, a very Woody one too — we have the religious fanatic, the unconventional crazy optimist. At its best it gives a mature and hopeful will to succeed together with others in an ordered world. Growth is comfortable if it is orderly.

This orderliness is the key to the connection between ♃ and Wood. But it is not the orderliness of a bus queue, nor a dull routine. It springs from what the Chinese call the Liver's function of maintaining a free flow of qi, ensuring harmonious circulation of energy. This means that when the Liver qi is healthy and unobstructed, all other types of energy flow smoothly, and mind and body on all levels integrate, with any excesses or deficiencies smoothed out, the congestion disseminated, the obstructions loosened.

Liver has been described as a general who excels in strategic planning: he not only determines and shapes the personality and how it projects itself smoothly in the world, but also copes with all the problems that get in the way, protecting and defending the organism. This defensive activity comes about through Liver's ability to store and release energy as required.

So any kind of disorder, be it emotional, spiritual or physical, if it involves blockage of free-flowing qi, is a responsibility of Liver energy. There are very few diseases where Liver is not affected.

Functions of Liver

1. Liver stores the blood

This means that it regulates the quantity and quality of fluids, particularly blood, in circulation at any time. When we are active, more blood is needed. When we rest or sleep, blood returns to its store, which in Chinese physiological terms is the liver. So if, for example, it fails to store the blood, then during sleep the blood will be circulating too much, and we shall not enjoy quiet repose; instead we shall have nightmares or bad dreams. We shall wake up, because blood is too near the surface. At night, blood should be at the centre, acting as an anchor for us. Without that anchor, we drift towards wakefulness.

Wood is a rising, increasing energy. Thus inefficient Liver Blood gives a pale face, blurred vision, possibly with floaters in the eyes, or dry eyes, or eye muscle spasms (tics) and giddiness in standing up suddenly. Liver Blood is the nourishing yin aspect of Liver; and as Liver governs anything that gets us going and on the move, Liver Blood nourishes our muscles and tendons. If poorly nourished by Liver Blood, muscles get cramps, numbness and weakness, with joints that are stiff to move. (The size and consistency of our flesh and muscles is, however, not Liver's responsibility, but that of Spleen. So wasted muscles due to deficient Spleen may retain movement and response, but lack underlying strength. The Liver Blood deficiency means that even a healthy and well-kept muscle lacks 'go' and elasticity.)

The Liver is traditionally associated with our nails; if Liver Blood is deficient these become dry and cracked, and break easily.

The other main blood movement that comes (partly) under Liver is menstruation, from menarche to menopause. This regular monthly cycle is required to make space in the womb. Amenorrhoea, or very scanty periods, is often due to deficient Liver. Lack of periods may be due either to 'stuck Liver', the inability of the Liver to trigger off a period, or to a deficiency of Liver Blood — so the blood is scanty or pale. Periods that drag on and on may also be due to a Liver that cannot recommence the cycle, a Liver qi problem. (The action of the contraceptive pill on menstruation is often to take over, then supplant, Liver's action. Many of the side-effects of this drug are related to Liver malfunction. For example, if there is a weak Liver in the first place, or a Liver weakened by prolonged use of contraceptives, there can arise many psychological and emotional problems; increase of weight, water retention; reduction in sexual appetite; allergies. When use of the drug ceases, Liver may be unable to recommence the menstrual cycle, and may cause a heavy feeling of depression, both physically and mentally.)

The Blood is an important residence of our personality and, if upset, we suffer disturbances of character, as anyone who has suffered a haemorrhage knows: we panic as our blood flows away. After giving birth to a baby, a mother frequently gets upset and depressed. In traditional Chinese medicine this is due to suffering the loss of a major part of herself, and her consequent inability to receive proper nourishment through the Blood until control of the new situation is reasserted. The child has been part of the mother, both sharing the same blood and contributing to it. How sad for both if the child is not breast-fed, promptly and for some months, because at least the mutual contact then remains to some extent. But from birth onwards, the mother receives no physical contribution to her blood from the child, hence her loss. She has to begin again as a person, and the Liver governs her ability.

2. Liver keeps qi flowing smoothly
It disperses excess and harmonizes the whole vitality. When it fails, Liver qi stagnates, or gets 'Stuck'. The importance of this cannot be over-emphasized. It acts in three main ways: emotional; in other organs and channels; and through the Gall Bladder. These are dealt with below.

Emotional
In the West, the predominant number of complaints in well-fed and housed societies derive from emotional disharmony: psychosomatic disease, where we cannot live contentedly with others or with ourselves.

The emotion associated with frustrated Liver function is anger, a natural energy of life. It clears us out. But in civilized society, we pay the price for suppressing it. We get depressed, stubborn, obstinate or temperamental. In particular, we lose an ability to experience other emotions freely: we get stuck into our grief, or our fear, our hysterical laughter, our apathy or worry. What is happening is that the Liver is failing to disperse our stuck emotional state. Hence our bursts of oversensitivity, brooding lack of tranquillity, hypochondria and depression.

This is not to say that these states are unnatural in themselves. But when our experience of them is prolonged, our Liver loses its ability to free us from their emotional burden. We cannot think our way out of it either — the Liver is our planner too. So we are 'stuck'; 'stuck Liver' means temperamental people.

People with good Liver function know how to get themselves well, and are less frequent visitors to the therapists; so if the charts in this book seem to point often to weak Livers — this is how it is. Those with good Livers don't turn up so much! (From a strictly commercial point of view, the drug companies have a big incentive to keep their drugs on the market. Drugs have a major effect on the Liver, and in the long term weaken it. The more drugs taken, whether social or medicinal or contraceptive, the greater the likelihood of a weak Liver, with consequent hypochondria: a wonderful commercial vicious circle.)

Since the Liver's function is to ease the flow of qi, there is no such thing as deficient Liver qi, though there may be deficiencies of qi in one place balanced by excesses of qi in others (hot head, cold feet for example). Actual total deficiency of vitality comes from other organs, Spleen and Kidney especially. Many people who think they are always tired or without energy are nothing of the sort — assuming they eat and sleep enough, of course. The telltale symptoms are those of depression and irascibility. A really tired person lacks the ability to be depressed or angry — he just needs rest and food. (Nervous anxiety and tiredness is more a symptom of Heart-Kidney deficiency, but it can come from a stuck Liver.) So where there seems to be no special emotional 'stuckness', the Liver is probably not involved.

There is one apparent exception to this general rule, and one that is common in Britain. There is a large class of individuals who were taught not to show any emotions other than those of polite pleasure or mild concern. They are frequently taken advantage of. They end up with many physical symptoms, usually associated with Liver or Gall Bladder problems, but they do not seem to have the expected emotion. Poor at self-defence and aggression, they lack anger. Their bodies show the anger that they are unable to feel. Sometimes it is very hard for these individuals to know what they feel at all. But they can become deeply depressed and sad, although unable to admit it. Life seems to pass them by; they become hopeless, and lose interest in variety. If they cry, they cry alone. If anything, they seem sad or grieving, at least from the sounds of their voices. Not infrequently, they hold quite irrational grudges and hates for those who have taken advantage of them and caused them offence. But all this is hidden. They find great difficulty in retaliating openly, and they may actually avoid sympathy. They prefer to work in safe places, out of the public eye, for large organizations where their loyalty is not questioned. In astrological terms, their 12th houses are usually occupied.

A stuck Liver is usually easy to diagnose. To treat it successfully depends on the depth and chronicity of the malaise. If very chronic and deep-seated, acupuncture, for example, will have a remarkably soothing effect, but the underlying reasons need to be investigated, and other therapies may at times be more appropriate, as, too, will education. (Most people who are unemployed for any length of time know what a stuck Liver feels like. If they cannot find a job or use their time and energy in some other creative or fulfilling way they will remain stuck. No amount of acupuncture will cure them; their life situation is the problem.) At the same time the therapist needs to be aware of his own psychological state, and able to help his patients in spite of it, if below par that day!

If our Liver cannot smooth the progress of our life, we suffer from setbacks and upsets. Life and health do not proceed as we would wish; we cannot rely on energy being there when we need it. We vacillate: we decide, then change our minds. We cannot commit ourselves. We waste time and energy. Our vitality fluctuates.

Qi in other organs and channels

Without a smooth flow of qi throughout the body, the qi gets obstructed and diverts its energy elsewhere, interfering with other functions either in the organs or along the channels.

The liver is placed in the middle 'chou' or middle 'burning space' of the body, the area bounded beneath by a horizontal line through the umbilicus and above by the diaphragm, so it is well placed to cause maximum disruption to the digestive system, and may also interfere with the respiratory system, for example.

Digestive system (Spleen-Stomach) middle and lower chou

'Wood over-acts on Earth.' This is experienced as various symptoms, varying from difficulty in swallowing food, or aversion to it, to ravenous hunger despite satiety. More commonly we find nausea, vomiting, belching, flatulence, epigastric pain, indigestion, stuffy chest, distension, bloating, the feeling of a mass in the abdomen, abdominal noises and constipation; also a bitter taste in the mouth and signs of jaundice. If qi fails to flow smoothly for too long, we get ulcers and tumours. Typically Liver qi indigestion is lessened by belching.

All these have to do with spasms, paralysis and reversed peristalsis, signs of stuck Liver qi 'on the prowl'.

The digestive system in women includes their breasts and the menstrual cycle. Qi disharmony gives pre-menstrual tension, hard, swollen and painful breasts and abdomen, pre-menstrual gains in weight, oedema and irregular periods. The menstruation itself may be heavy or light depending, for example, on whether there is Heat in the Blood, or deficient qi, both of which might give profuse bleeding but for quite different reasons; and on whether there is deficient Blood or perhaps coagulated Blood, each of which under different circumstances might give scanty bleeding.

If qi attacks upwards to the throat, we get difficulty swallowing due to a sensation in the throat which the Chinese call 'plumstone in the throat'. Typically this occurs when self-conscious, or thinking about problems, and improves when relaxed. This is another instance of Liver qi 'tightening up', here preventing smooth progress of food.

Upper chou
The Liver meridian passes from the hypochondorium, through the diaphragm and chest, in all of which areas stuck qi can show as distension and difficulty in breathing. Sighing is a natural release of obstructed qi, occurring when we are frustrated. Difficult breathing, hay fever, asthma, and many feelings of tightness, fullness and stuffiness in the chest come from stuck qi. Stuck qi in the diaphragm causes hiccups (though this is not their only cause).

It should be noted first, that in practice not all the mentioned symptoms occur at the same time! Secondly, organic changes such as enlargement of the liver, hepatitis and cirrhosis can also lead to these manifestations, as can certain other syndromes in Chinese pathology.

Blood
Stuck Liver qi often affects the Blood, producing either stagnation and the build-up of tumours and masses under the skin — often along the course of the Liver channel — or a tendency to haemorr-

hage or psoriasis. (But there are usually other contributory causes also.) Hot Blood injures the meridian and often spills outwards, making the blood circulate wildly — almost as if it were on the boil. Symptoms include bleeding, rashes (e.g. scarlet fever and measles), hives, fever, irritability, thirst and a feeling of heat — as if hurting. Menstrual signs are a heavy flow that may come early (the heat forces it through early) and pain before the period, that is worse for rubbing. For a fuller discussion of Blood, see page 132.

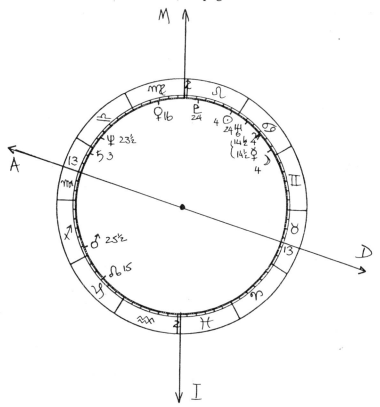

Chart 2. Female, 29.

Case 2: Female, 29
Case 2 came with eczema worse in winter, especially of the right hand, that swelled, went red, followed by little blisters under the skin that itched and burned intolerably, making her very irritable. She had an allergy to dust of various origins that made her eyes stream, with much yawning, sneezing, itchy skin and facial swelling. Eyes were

always tired, worse for strong light and felt as if bursting. Neck glands were swollen all the time. She got bad pre-menstrual tension with headaches in the occipital area that seemed to be bursting. Her periods were painful but scanty, blood fresh red with deep red clots. She had ileocaecal area distension occasionally. She was averse to oily fish, strawberries and red wine. Her neck was usually rigid. She got catarrh with green lumps. Generally she was better at 11 a.m. and worst between 4 p.m. and 7 p.m., when she got a headache in her right temple. Her job overworked her; she was, she said, 'under great stress', 'neurotic' and 'anxious about everything'. She hated crowds and shops — there was too much bustle. She seemed to be on the thin line where she knew quite clearly that she was going to lose control; she spoke in a strained voice but quietly, with very intelligent probing questions, but it seemed that only massive self-control was holding her together. She loved sleeping, but it did not refresh her. She preferred drinking to eating; lots of tea and white wine in particular. Even in the coldest weather in Scotland she never felt cold air, and wore just one layer of clothing.

Her chart shows a powerful personality (Ascendant ♏, ☉ and ruler ♇ in ♌, ♂ in ♐, with considerable administrative ability (♏, ♌ and four planets in ♋ 8/9 houses) a tendency to work for others, possibly to her own disadvantage, perhaps because of difficulty communicating with her parents at an early age, with sense of guilt (☉ □ ♄$_{12}$, ☽ △ ♄$_{12}$), and great sensitivity used on others' behalf, with artistic sensibility (♏ + ♋). The outstanding planet is ♂, alone in its hemisphere, giving her a fairly pugnacious and aggressive attitude, with strong powers of perseverance, and a need to explore new horizons. Although good at routine work, she will want to keep moving on until she meets either an individual or a challenge stronger than herself that gives her a hope of eventual success but does not frighten her.

That strong ♂, in traditional Chinese medicine, points immediately to a Fire problem, quite possibly one of overheating, overworking or over-sensualizing. Cancer planets suggest absorption and dietary problems, and the strong emphasis on ♃ throughout the chart (e.g. part ruler ♂ in ♐, part ruler ♇ and ☉ in 9th house, ♃ ☌ ☿ △ A, and the lack of compensating strength in ♄$_{12}$) gives a tendency to change, movement, new ideas and plans that will brook little interference, yet will, because of the position of ♄, not enable her sufficiently to consolidate her strength in Earth. Earth governs digestion, absorption and production of qi and Blood. Of qi she will have little shortage — witness the ♂, ☉ + ♇ and ♃ △ A. But her Blood could easily be unruly and there is likely to be considerable strain on her kidneys, governed by ☿ in traditional Chinese medicine.

So we have a picture of someone who overworks and overheats and over-responds (e.g. allergies) from a predominance of ♃ and ♂, Wood and Fire phase, without a sufficient balance from a stabilizing ♄, Earth. She will always tend to live life to the maximum — not an uncommon Scorpionic trait — which strains her Water energy.

At the time of her consultation, the diagnosis was self-evident, and the chart was erected only when this book was being written. The unknown factor was the direct cause of her problems, which she said had been developing for almost twelve years (the ♃ cycle). She was asked where she had holidayed twelve years before, and she remembered a July holiday in the Mediterranean, when she had sunbathed on the beach without a towel between skin and hot sand. One of the classic causes of heat in the Blood due to 'perverse evil of (summer) heat' entering straight into the blood is sitting on hot, sunbaked rocks. Nowadays the problem also occurs in, for example, children who sit on hot radiators in winter or, as in this case, those who lie on bare sand. (Those who sit on hot radiators do not of course always get Heat in the Blood! But their bodies will get Heat somewhere, and often it particularly affects the lower chou, the area underneath the umbilicus, producing Heat symptoms there, notably Hot-type diarrhoea — the urgent kind!) In this case the patient exposed both surfaces of the body to the Heat: radiant from above, direct from underneath, so there may or may not also have been other temporary signs of Heat. These often occur on summer holidays in hot climates for those from northern climates who eat or drink very Heating-type fare, and then wonder why they experience Hot-type digestive disturbances.

Analysing her problem in traditional Chinese medicine: the rash, feeling of heat, thirst, swollen glands, face, pre-menstrual tension, headaches, aversion to heat-producing foods are directly attributable to Heat in the Blood. The right-sidedness of her symptoms is due to this being the side on which Liver imbalances occur most often. Heat rises, so causing the streaming eyes and sneezing. Yawning is due to the Kidney energy (☿) being too weak to hold the qi sent down to it by the Lungs. Tired eyes, worse for light, indicate a weakness in Liver Blood. There are many Liver qi stuck syndromes: the pre-menstrual tension, state of frustration derived from overwork, ileocaecal area bloating, hatred of crowds and irritability. There are also hints of the beginnings of a Heart-Kidney polarity imbalance, with the overemphasis on Fire and underemphasis on the calm relaxation and rest of Earth (♄) and Water (☿), as evidenced by her general anxiety, barely held state of self-control and feeling best at 11 a.m. (the start of the Heart two-hour period; see Chapter 10). Kidney overstrain by Liver shows up in neck rigidity, occipital headaches pre-menstrually (occiput is traversed by the Bladder meridian) and tiredness at 4-7 p.m. (Water time). There were signs of deficient Blood: her menses were scanty, and she was beginning to panic. However, all was not lost (!) as the menstrual blood had good colour; but deep red clots pointed to stagnant qi.

Overall, there is a picture of someone whose way of living tends to send energy upwards to the head — e.g. from mental strain and worry — whose body is afflicted with Heat, which also sends energy upwards and disturbs harmonious dispersion of excess by the Liver. Simplified, the diagnosis was: Heat in Blood disturbing Liver function and shen.

(For those astrologers who collect associations, the dust to which she was allergic was that of horse (♃) and that found in French homes; i.e. the dust of foreign places (♃)!)

This is a case where an underlying Wood emphasis and an invading perverse evil contrived to ruin a patient's health. Acupuncture treatment to reduce the Heat in the Blood, smooth the Liver and regulate Heart-Kidney energy produced a great improvement. However, the stresses of her job gave her much mental worry and she continued to experience catarrh. She was not enjoying her work, and eventually applied for an easier job in another town: this seemed to be the right decision, symbolized by a better ♃-♄ balance, which occurred when T♄ entered the 1st house. The original Mediterranean holiday occurred when ♂ was transiting natal ☉, ruler ♇ in ♌, and progressed ☉♌ was opposition P ☽ ♒, itself a symbol of yang versus yin, or Heat versus Cold.

Gall Bladder, bile secretion and excretion
A small but important function of the Liver. The Gall Bladder meridian and energy are involved too, but the Liver energy is responsible for smooth flow of bile into the intestine.

3. Liver nourishes, or dominates, the tendons
The tendons are the seat of the springiness that gets us moving and gives us resilience, and this is perhaps why they are governed by the Liver. But muscles also are controlled by the Liver. However,

nourishment of muscles in general is governed by the Spleen and Stomach.

The distinction may seem confusing. Broadly speaking, if our muscles are undernourished, perhaps because we eat poorly or cannot digest and use food properly, then the Stomach/Spleen energy is responsible. But if, despite good food, we suffer from flat feet, fallen arches, pulled muscles and lack of resilient 'give' on a physical level (and, probably, on an emotional level too) then the Liver Blood is deficient.

The same goes for cramps and paralysis (which can of course have other causes, however).

In health, the yin part of Liver function, its Blood, gives smooth normal muscle contraction and relaxation, with strength and flexibility. If insufficient, we get spasms, numbness and poor mobility.

So Spleen governs a muscle's substance; Liver governs its function, its mobility, its relaxed alertness.

4. Liver 'opens' into the eyes

All the organs influence the eyes to some extent, but the Liver is predominant, governing clarity of vision and movement of the eyes. In sleep we close our eyes: Liver Blood is no longer needed to nourish them. Continually tired eyes suggest deficient Liver Blood. Nervous tics round the eyes also point to Liver: associated with Wind, a tic is a trapped bit of Wind, though it is probably also due to deficient yin, or Blood.

5. Liver governs physical endurance

Before discussing this, it must be said that the energy of Spleen, Stomach and Kidney (Earth and Water) also play an important part here. But the Liver rallies the forces; so if we cannot decide on our plans for the future, the Liver energy is not acting properly. (It may also upset control in other areas, such as mouth or nose, with mouth left half-open, dribbling and urine flow uncontrolled. This is the reason why epileptics often have urinary dysfunction even when not 'en grand mal'.)

The defensive energy of the body comes from several sources, but in the first instance it comes from the Lungs, which rule the skin. But the Liver mobilizes this defensive energy. If we catch a cold, then the Liver has failed in its purpose. It is not surprising that most people who get depressed (= depressed Liver qi) also catch colds.

When we grow tired, the Liver energy is depleted — our reserves have run out. The only way to restore them is by rest and food. But the Liver decides our ability to recover energy after fatigue. Wood in the phase diagram occupies the position after Water, where energy is arising. So if we cannot wake up in the morning, or if we do not feel refreshed in spite of a fairly good sleep, then one strong possibility is that Liver qi is not functioning properly.

6. Liver controls the lower chou
(or lower abdomen, the space inferior to the umbilicus)
This control is shared with the Kidneys, e.g.:

1. the functions of the large intestine and the rectum in a smooth flow of faeces;
2. the sexual energy and physical condition of the genitals;
3. ovulation and menstruation and conception.

In terms of sexual energy, it is the ability to get interested in the opposite sex that is meant, on the emotional and physical levels; equally, the timing in the body that decides when to ovulate, to menstruate, and to embark on conception. Both sexual response and the menstrual cycle are a readying of the body, rallying itself for a new departure (or arrival!) in life. They signify an aspect of 'Waking'. A chart of impotency is discussed under ☿, Chapter 5 (Chart 5).

Syndromes of Liver
The main syndromes of Liver are:

1. Liver qi stuck;
2. Liver-Blood deficiency;
3. Hyperactive Liver yang;
4. Liver Fire ascending;
5. Liver Wind stirring;
6. Damp Heat in Liver and Gall Bladder; ⎫
7. Cold stagnates in Liver channel.   ⎬ not discussed here.
                                            ⎭

There are many books that describe these syndromes in careful detail. As stuck Liver and Liver Blood deficiency have already been discussed, at the risk of offending other practitioners I shall describe briefly together hyperactive Liver yang, Liver Fire ascending and Liver Wind stirring, each of which is an aspect of one sub-picture. In each case the picture is energy rising upwards, although the causes are different, as follows.

1. *Liver yang hyperactive*
   This arises from Liver yin deficiency (which itself arises either from Liver Blood deficiency or Kidney yin deficiency).

2. *Liver Fire Ascending*
   This comes either from chronic Liver qi stagnation, or from an already 'heated Liver' being sparked into Fire by a sudden rage, or a heavy alcoholic drinking bout, or even smoking. (Alcohol or cigarettes are probably being taken to smooth tension, which they do in the short term. Unfortunately, alcohol in particular has a longer-term heating effect on the Blood, whereas cigarettes mainly stimulate Lungs to send qi down to the kidneys, reinforcing Kidney function including Kidney yin, so temporarily cooling the Liver Heat. They also stimulate Kidney yang, and Heart yang, which is why smokers need cigarettes to keep warm. Unfortunately, in the long term this heating function is eroded, and smokers suffer increasingly poor circulation, as in Reynaud's syndrome. Alcoholics on the other hand have a tendency to Heat in the Blood, so feel hot most of the time. In the short term, therefore, both alcohol and cigarettes have a warming effect, though they may relax, but for different reasons.)

3. *Liver Wind stirring*
   The Wind meant here is what is termed an internal evil, and is neither caused by nor related to diseases due to external perverse Wind. However, that said, its characteristics are very windy! It is caused by:
   (a) an acute excessive Liver Fire ascending, the blaze of which creates a 'draught' of Wind;
   (b) hyperactive Liver yang being so powerful that it creates a wake and pulls the Wind up after it;
   (c) Blood deficiency, where the deficiency is such that one imagines bubbles of emptiness creating a vacuum into which the Wind rushes.

For our purposes, the key symptoms are:

Irritability.
Headaches that are bursting and throbbing.
Dry mouth and throat. Thirst.
Sleeplessness.

Plus

Liver Yang	Liver Fire	Liver Wind
Dizziness	Red face	Shaking, trembling
Poor memory	Eyes bloodshot	Tic
Cramps	Eyes swollen	Numbness
Numbness	Sudden tinnitus,	Seizures
Noises in the ears	even deafness	Dizziness
Sinus problems	Bile in the mouth	Loss of consciousness
Blurred vision	Bleeding nose or	
Tired eyes	gums, or vomiting	
	blood	
	Constipation with	
	dry stools and	
	dark urine	

The increasing severity of these syndromes can be seen by reading from left to right. In Liver yang and Liver Wind there is some deficiency, leading to dizziness, numbness and forgetfulness. In Liver Fire, the picture is just one of excess, bursting upwards. In Western terms these are syndromes such as insomnia, hypertension, migraine, neurosis, stomach ulcers, menopausal problems, many eye and ear diseases and glaucoma, as well as a multitude of complaints such as 'burnt tongue', alcoholism, low back problems (the yin deficient part of the syndrome), heartburn, cracking joints, epilepsy, sexual problems, neck and shoulder tension and pain.

The remaining syndromes not discussed here (Damp Heat and Cold Stagnation) are important in themselves but partly discussed elsewhere under 'Damp Heat' and 'Cold' respectively.

The main aim here is to give an idea of the energy represented primarily by ♃ in the birth chart, and of the ways it causes disease when obstructed.

Paths of Wood Phase Meridians

The Gall Bladder channel originates from the outer canthus of the eye, rises to the corner of the forehead, runs round posterior to the ear, back over the side of the head to a point on the forehead above the eye, then back again over the side of the head to the side of the neck and along the shoulder. It therefore covers a large part of the side of the head. There are branches from the channel into the ear, to the seventh cervical vertebra, and to the cheeks. The main channel runs down the side of the chest, through the free ends of the floating ribs to the hip region, where it meets the internal pathway which has descended from the neck region through diaphragm, liver and gall bladder and hypochondrial region to a point near the femoral artery in the groin. It skirts the margin of the pubic hair and then goes deep into the hip.

From the deep muscles of the hip it descends the thigh along its lateral aspect, continuing along the lateral aspect of the leg to a point anterior to the external malleolus; thence to the fourth toe, sending a branch to the big toe, where it becomes the Liver meridian.

The Liver channel runs from the big toe along the dorsum of the foot, up the medial aspect of the shin and thigh to the pubic region, where it curves around the external genitalia, entering the lower abdomen, ascending to curve round the stomach, and enters liver and gall bladder organs. It continues upwards through the diaphragm, with branches to costal and hypochondriac regions, then along the back of the throat to the nasopharynx and eye system, emerging finally from the forehead to end on the vertex.

Jupiter is known by astrologers to have associations with several points along this channel such as the foot (Pisces), thigh (Sagittarius) and liver. Traditional Chinese medicine adds an important array of possible pain sites, notably the eyes, side of head, and neck region lateral to the trapezius muscles. Liver problems often occur in the shoulder area (tension), down the sides of the chest and in the sides and iliac fossa of the abdomen.

The hip is the next major area. A vast number of individuals suffering from sciatica and hip joint difficulty are suffering from Wood type problems: hip replacements occur very often in those who have either stuck Liver, or deficient Liver yin as they grow older.

The position of Jupiter in the charts of individuals with migraine — with its eye disturbances, unilateral headache and nausea — is nearly always prominent.

Case 3: Female, 82

Chart 3 is of someone who suffered from stuck Liver all her life. Periodically it imploded into Liver Fire and Wind. Her presenting complaints were tension, low backache, poor sleep — particularly bad about 3 a.m. to 5 a.m., when she woke 'paralysed'. Of rare ability and insight, she was quite overcome by what she knew were quite illogical, not to say insane, likes and dislikes for her fellow man. She was unable to show anger, though she could be a little short with people, feeling acutely guilty afterwards. Early life had been marred by jealousy, fear and a mother who was unable to defend her children from the insane rages of their father. The whole family was artistically gifted. She had undergone many years of analysis.

The strong oppositions and conjunctions in the chart point to intensity, as does the Ascendant ♏. How frequently ♏ Ascendants occur in the charts of those who must control their environments! (To compensate for their deep insecurity and to hide from others' probings of their fears and guilts?) In the chart, the tightest group of planets is ☽ ☌ ♄ ☍ ♇, signalling personal inadequacy and jealousy, and a lifelong mental tension. (Moon and Saturn both relate to Earth, and the ability to think things over steadily. They also relate to the gastro-intestinal tract: seldom was she other than constipated.) As is to be suggested later, ♅ is a planet closely related to Wood, and she was a very temperamental person. She had good powers of self-expression, a good eye and a precise mind (☿ ☌ ♂). The highest planet in the chart, alone and a singleton, is ♃. She had travelled widely and was well-educated. She had done much teaching of a therapeutic nature. At one time famous, it bothered her that she had never really made her name again. She preferred independence. She suffered acute depression.

Whenever we see squares and oppositions, we think of 'tension', which is a Liver word. There was little outlet for this patient's frustration, and as she grew older, her body less able to carry her around, the tensions worsened. One day she had a cerebral hae-morrhage affecting the right side of her body, the Liver side, another example of the free yang energy demolishing the yin — right side. The transits and progressed positions at the time of stroke are numerous, but the main ones are PM = 10° ♐; T♇ = 26½° ♎; T♅ = 2½° ♐; T♃ = 5° ♏; T♂ = 5° ♎ (= ♃/♅); T☽ was in early ♐; T♀ = 8° ♒.

In this chart, ♃ is in a Fire sign and in its own house, so one would expect its effect to be at least partly beneficial. She was very tall, and she had a comfortable inheritance. But whilst she lived on to a considerable age — way past her stroke — Jupiter's effect is tightly constrained by the energy of ☿ ☌ ♂. We see here the rulers of three connecting phases, Water, Wood and Fire, closely intertwined into an aspect of tension. Many ☿ ☌ ♂ types have quick tongues, and the strength of ♃ seems to have accentuated that tension. What in another chart would have led to a feeling of belonging, comfort with herself and calm reflection (aspects of ☽ and ♄ at their best) are impossible here. The past (☽ and ♄) is tied too closely to feelings

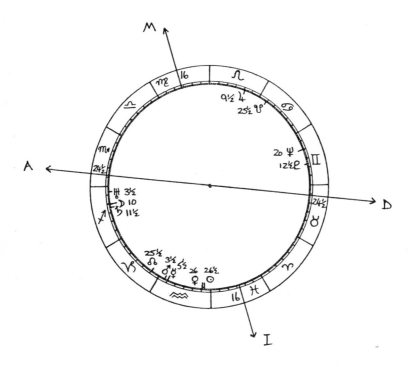

Chart 3. Female, 82.

of jealousy and suspicion (♇) about her family by opposition, so she lacked a tempering influence on the angry tensions of the opposition from ♃ to ☿ ♂.

The remaining phase energy of ♀ which one might have expected to give balance, is rendered too yang by conjunction with ☉.

Planets conjunct the sun are said to be combust: in at least the cases of ☿ and ♀, their effect is to some extent less strong. Using the phase diagram we can see why: the sun symbolizes the energy of life, yang, qi. Venus and Mercury are associated with yin phases, and their ability to produce yin effects is therefore to some extent lost by conjunction with the most yang symbol of all. The same occurs to a lesser extent in ♂ conjunctions with the yin phase planets. (For further discussion see Chapter 8.)

3.

MARS ♂

Mars represents activity in which there is an element of self-assertion, of enterprise and impulse. It is the enjoyment of independent self-expression, whether emotional, sensual, aggressive, initiatory or obstinate. It is our desire for action and self-revelation; our drive for results and our satisfaction in identifying ourselves with these results. It is how we enjoy excitement, our liking for power, and how we relish our sexual and physical urges. It is the way we luxuriate in self-gratification. In the chart it is how we take pleasure in selfish activity, impressing ourselves on those around us. It symbolizes man's sexuality, how he revels in his manhood.

No wonder it has a bad reputation. Selfishness is usually at someone else's cost, and seen as impatient, destructive and uncaring. Greed, lust and all the host of character defects that man points at his fellow come under its domain, at least in the sensuous display of their need. There is nothing enigmatic or hidden about Mars.

How can we relate this to the Fire phase, and to the energies that relate primarily to Fire of the Heart, Small Intestine and Pericardium meridian? Let us take Heart and Pericardium together, and leave Small Intestine aside for the moment.

These are the parts of ourselves that open to others when we have something deep to share. If in love, we speak from the heart, yet being in love ties us closely to need for the loved one. At more refined levels, our love is shared, and the other person's life can become more important than our own; we expand our feelings to include another, and move out from ourselves. The expression of our own sunny self-enjoyment shines out on others. If the Sun represents the urge to live, Mars is its most energetic direct manifestation. So ♂ is how we play, though ☉ gives us our playfulness. An easy Mars gives a direct expression of our needs. It allows us to be open and direct. Our emotions flow freely; we say what we want and we feel it as we say it. (The consequences of our action are another matter!) Many religions teach this direct simplicity as being healthy. Those who surround their lives and motives with craft, guile, with moral imperatives and condemnations — the oughts and shoulds — cannot express themselves in this naive, childish and free way.

The Fire phase is the high noon of our energy, the part of life that revels in display, colour, laughter and enjoyment; it is also the part representing falling in love, mixing in joyful co-operation with another. It is the time of fun, enjoyment, good things, pleasure and success, praising others and being praised ourselves. We work for money so as to be able to live, but more, to enjoy ourselves. It is the reason we hope to win at lotteries; we wish to shine. At a higher level it is a refined, non-egotistic sharing, and at still higher levels it is pure love and joyful awareness of an interconnectedness between all things, the light that may be hidden but which makes things as they are.

Mars is ruler of Aries, known for its aggressive self-interest. It also rules Scorpio, another symbol for which is the Eagle which flies higher than any of the other signs of the Zodiac. Mars encompasses both saint and sinner, both pioneer and saviour. When Mars works purely for itself, then the light does not shine outwards, and we see darkness, selfishness and the reasons for giving the planet its traditional evil classification; it is thus when we seek gratification of our desires at the expense of others. Not so when we direct our energy outwards to improve the lot of all life. We may be just as individualistic and aggressive and difficult, but we are driven by a moral imperative higher than ourselves, and Heat, traditionally associated with Mars, now warms our companions. This is where we can relate Mars and Fire phase in traditional Chinese medicine. The Fire phase contains the Heart and Pericardium which relate to joy and love and which, in the case of the Heart, fulfils the role of Sovereign Ruler from whom there emanates a directing influence and a pure insight and awareness. The Heart governs integrity of individuality. It represents the 'Heart of our personality'. (It is not the life force of the personality itself, nor the directing soul behind our life: that supreme monarch traditionally resides in the upper 'field of cinnabar' approximately one inch behind the point midway between the eyes. But the Heart Official is Sovereign Prince to that Emperor.)

Functions of Heart

1. Heart 'controls and governs' the blood, blood vessels and pulse
Without blood there is no life. Without a pulse, there is no blood.

So Blood depends on the Heart. Circulation of blood gives a consistent base for life (circulation here includes lymphatic drainage), as it nourishes every part of the body. Circulation proceeds through the networks of arteries, capillaries and veins. When there is sufficient blood supply and a healthy circulation, we have a good complexion and a potent vitality.

The Heart's role in governing Blood is important because the Blood (and yin) are where *shen* (the spirit) resides.

To get a limited idea of the Heart's role here, consider what happens when we bruise, and blood escapes from the capillaries into surrounding flesh, which swells. The shock of a major bruise, or accident, affects the mind — we go into shock; blood pressure falls and heartbeat rate changes. Shock is one case where the Blood ceases to be a residence of the spirit, which cannot then function properly.

2. Heart houses the shen

There is no easy way to describe shen, but it is the first thing that an experienced practitioner of any kind of medicine looks for. It appears as an alert, lively responsiveness to life, a sparkle in the eye, an ability to create, to work, to act. Without it we lack spirit, nerve and 'go', and no matter how trifling our disease, we shall be hard to cure. But even someone with a terminal cancer can have good shen and be able to create situations where he can enjoy life, or what remains of it for him. Shen contains daring and the enjoyment of challenge.

But it also implies awareness, memory and our ability to think. Depression can come from the Heart as well as from Liver and Lung. But whereas in the case of the Liver the depression is from obstruction, from the Heart it is from loss of enjoyment of life.

Because the Heart is the acting prince in control of the body, he is ultimately responsible for everything in the body, so must be considered as a possible contributory cause wherever there is a major imbalance in vitality, noticeably as regards yin and yang.

It is always dangerous to make comparisons with Western medicine, but the Heart function certainly bears a strong relationship to the central nervous system.

If the Heart fails to house the shen properly, we may dream during our sleep. Strange and even provocative though it may seem, an entirely healthy Heart gives a restful, unworried and dream-free sleep. (Perhaps we should say that no dreams are remembered — but this is not what the Chinese say!) A stronger indication is insomnia, with many dreams, and absentmindedness which, as the situation worsens, leads to neurosis, hypertension, mental disorders, palpitations and delirium; the shen is confused. Sleeping pills may suppress sleeplessness, but if long continued they do not give sleep as the Heart does not learn again how to house the shen.

3. Heart manifests in the complexion
If healthy, the face should be moist and rosy, with good texture and clarity. Consider the soft colour of the nun, who has striven with her soul for years and is at peace with herself. Never has she used cosmetics. Compare it with that of someone who drinks alcohol too much. He may have a vivid colour, but it is a sign of Heat. The Chinese call the face the 'Window of the Soul'!

4. Heart opens into the tongue — 'The Mirror of the Heart'

(a) Speech: a pure heart gives clear self-expression. If the Heart is troubled we get problems with our speech; we slur words or stutter. The tongue will not move to order.
(b) Taste: a healthy tongue — and Heart — can distinguish different tastes. Sometimes people with major traumatic memories that have given them sleepless nights for years, temporarily lose their ability to taste and smell as they begin to improve.
(c) The tongue's body is a reflection of the state of the Heart. Deep cracks, for instance, are one pointer towards Heart problems, especially if near the tip; so too is the colour red.

5. The Heart's fluid is sweat
This is not the sweat that comes from healthy exercise, but that which comes from anxiety and nervousness. Equally, spontaneous night sweating that is cold — i.e. one may be sweating freely but still feel cold — comes when Heart Blood or Heart yin is empty. Often this sweat has a scorched, burnt odour.

It should be said that the Pericardium meridian plays an important part in the Heart's work; some would say it has greater importance as regards relationships than the Heart, whereas the Heart has more to do with mental problems. There is a difference; but clinically they are treated often as being much the same. However, the following functions of the Heart are shared with those of the Pericardium.

6. Heart governs happiness and enjoyment
Love, compassion, passion, relationships, generosity and sharing;

the ebb and flow of warmth, including that generated by sexual relationships, the fun of music, dance and movement. Altruism and maturity.

But there is a wisdom here too that guides us out of hurtful relationships where we have wasted ourselves in unreciprocated outpourings of affection. And if we need the experience, this is the energy of desire that brings us together again, that makes us explore pastures new, that opens us to new influences.

Each of us needs the warmth of a joyful relationship. Deprivation starves our Fire phase energy so that we take less pleasure in life: life's embrace passes us by. We despair of loving contact, we see only futility, we become suicidal. Nothing brings us real fulfilment; we grow tired and exhausted in spirit, or angry and vindictive. We retreat into ourselves, afraid and isolated, and we surround ourselves with illogical worries and superstitious fears. We can fulfil ourselves neither emotionally nor sexually.

Alternatively we become obsessed with our own needs, possibly perverted, usually excessive in relation to necessity. We cling to old relationships, and we hurt. We have forgotten the joys of being human, as we 'lord' it over our peers.

We may go out of control; excess joy is hard to imagine as a threat to health, but that kind of laughter where energy is suspended at the point of inhalation, kept within, as in hysteria, damages the energy in the 'upper chou', especially that of the Heart.

Syndromes of Heart

1. Heart qi weak;
2. Heart yang weak;
3. Heart yin weak;
4. Heart Blood weak;
5. Heart Fire hyperactive;
6. Derangement of the mind;
7. Stagnation of Blood in the Heart.

For reasons of brevity, some of the above syndromes are combined in the following descriptions.

1. Heart qi weak — Heart yang weak
Weak Heart yang is developed in time out of a weak Heart qi. Weak Heart qi has two aspects:

(a) Weakness of Heart, which appears as palpitations.
(b) Weak qi, meaning lassitude, shortness of breath which is worse for exertion, a pale face and weak voice. The tongue is pale and swollen, and shows teeth marks round the sides. (Weak qi also crops up in syndromes of other zangfu.)

Heart yang weakness is superimposed on this, and since yang is warming and dispersing, weakness in yang leads to chilliness and cold extremities and a stuffy feeling in the chest. Yang qi weakness can cause Wei qi weakness, giving spontaneous sweating.

If Heart Yang becomes extremely weak, we get collapse, profuse sweating, coma and a fading thready pulse. Breathing is very weak. Purple lips and the feeble breathing are due to weak Heart yang being unable to move the Blood. Coma comes about because Heart yang has collapsed, and so cannot move the Blood properly, thus providing nowhere for the shen to reside.

The causes of these states are:

(a) Weakness of qi and yang due to prolonged illness, especially where there has been non-recovery from acute or chronic haemorrhage, as in internal bleeding and menorrhagia.
(b) Emotional problems, whether caused by melancholy, sadness, overthinking (i.e. worry) or fright, which hurt the shen.
(c) Over-use of yang due to overwork, too much sex, etc.

Note that because this is a situation of weak qi, palpitations are more likely to occur during activity, during daytime, because this is when qi is being strained, and has not the power to maintain a steady rhythm in the heart.

2. Weak Heart Blood

Palpitations, usually at night or when resting. During rest and sleep, the Blood is stored on the inside by the Liver. Shen seeks refuge in this Blood, but if it is deficient, cannot settle: so the Heart gives palpitations, often of the sudden 'bump' kind, or of a few quick beats in a row followed by a pause. Naturally, anxiety accompanies this. This happens more when lying flat. When sitting upright, the weight of gravity helps to compensate for the lack of 'mass' in the Blood.

Insomnia, restlessness and dream-disturbed sleep occur because the Blood provides no real home for the shen during sleep. Anxiety, absent-mindedness and poor memory occur because the shen has nowhere to store its experiences. Often there is a dull complexion

— not enough Blood! — and the tongue is pale for the same reason. The causes of weak Heart Blood are as follows.

(a) Here we have a nervous, sensitive and somewhat anaemic individual who is either very talkative and excitable or rather silent and averse to company, who has been a worrier for a long time. This state of anxiety has upset the Heart, which is no longer able to govern the Blood.

(b) The state can also come from poor food or eating habits, not uncommon in this kind of individual, even if he is a health faddist. The poor diet weakens the qi of the Spleen, one of whose jobs it is to turn food into Blood. Weak Blood leads to Weak Heart Blood.

(c) Any major blood loss will have the same effect; it can be through injury, internal bleeding or childbirth, which is a source of depression as mentioned under Liver Blood.

3. Weak Heart yin

This is an extension of Weak Heart Blood, although it can occur without some of the symptoms of weak Heart Blood.

Palpitations, poor memory, insomnia, dream-disturbed sleep, general restlessness and anxiety are symptoms shared with weak Heart Blood. In addition there is often a slight flush on the cheeks — known as a malar flush; a low fever or feeling of warmth or burning; spontaneous perspiration at night, and mild thirstiness.

These additional symptoms occur because yin, which is cooling and holds energy down, is weak, so yang appears to be strong, and weak signs of false yang excess appear, such as thirst and fever. The afternoon, a yin time, is when these symptoms become more noticeable, and yin deficient patients complain, for example, of a feeling of heat then, or a burning feeling in the upper parts of the body or head — e.g. the ears; or they may say that they only get thirsty in the late afternoon, or develop a flush then. The tongue is red and without covering: so here the yin deficiency has superimposed itself on the Blood deficiency which would normally give only a pale tongue. The tip of the tongue is sometimes the only part that goes red, and it may have a centre line crack right up to the tip.

The causes of Weak Heart yin are as follows.

(a) Emotional problems of long standing coupled with many years of hectic business activities — perhaps undertaken to fill the emotional vacuum. Someone who easily becomes anxious, though he may not show it — may even be unaware of it; who nurses old grievances deep down. Somewhere in this person is a deep melancholy: to avoid sinking into it he does far too much thinking and worrying, which damages the Heart, the residence of the spirit.

(b) In high fevers these symptoms may also appear, as the heat of the fever consumes the yin (cooling) fluids, giving the appearance of false yang; there is mental restlessness and sleeplessness. If the patient gets to this stage, although there will still be fever, he will start to feel the cold, and far from throwing off the bedclothes may actually desire more of them. Here the yang is beginning to get exhausted, having spent itself on 'boiling off' the yin fluids. So although yang is reduced, yin is still further depleted. If Kidney yin is already weak, then this will also exacerbate the situation.

4. Heart Fire hyperactive

Ulceration, swelling and pain of mouth and tongue, insomnia accompanied by a feverish sensation; face is flushed and there may be a bitter taste in the mouth; urine is painful, hot and a dark yellow; tongue is red with a yellow covering; mouth is thirsty and there is a general hurried restlessness.

These symptoms are signs of heat rising upwards in the body; ulceration, swollen mouth and tongue, etc., are symptoms that do not appear in deficiency. Here the face is flushed red; in deficiency it is pale with just a 'malar flush', worse in the afternoon. Here the redness is present at all times, and covers nose, cheeks and lips — the whole face, and ears too sometimes. The patient complains of feverishness and hot sensations.

If this syndrome appears on its own, there will be no palpitations; so why do we associate it with the Heart and not with the Liver? (See Liver Fire ascending, which also has red face, thirst, bitter taste and yellow urine.)

The Heart is associated with the tongue, which is ulcerated. It is also associated, or paired with, the Small Intestine meridian, which has a very close relationship with the Bladder meridian. The heat in the Heart passes through to the Bladder, causing painful burning urination. An important distinguishing feature is the temper: in Liver Fire there is a definite instability and a very short fuse on a nasty temper, which is much less marked in Heart Fire; but in Heart Fire there is usually a history of intense worry or anxiety. Liver Fire rises to the top of the head, with very painful headaches and red eyes, and gives nose-bleeds, noises in the ears, bleeding gums and a vomiting of blood. In Heart Fire, the only blood — if any — appears in the urine.

However, that being said, the causes of Liver Fire and Heart Fire are often quite similar, in that they can both arise from a long period of worry and depression which have repressed qi. This stagnant qi then suddenly explodes into Fire. Equally Liver Fire can also cause Heart Fire (see the phase diagram).

5. Derangement of the mind

There are many symptoms under this syndrome, which itself contains several distinct aspects, too detailed to discuss here. The main symptoms are mental depression, dullness of mind, muttering to oneself, weeping and laughing without apparent reason, incoherent speech, even mania, and crazy, rash behaviour. These can develop into unconsciouness, stupor and coma. Tongue colour is red, with a coating that may be thick and yellow.

Causes are normally either mental irritation depressing the Heart, or persistent high fever which forces 'Heat into the Pericardium', the area around the heart. Another cause is too much greasy food or alcohol both of which have a heating effect.

The reason these are associated with the Heart is that the mind — governed by Heart — is confused, so shen is disturbed. In terms of Chinese pathology, mucus or phlegm and Fire obstruct or 'mist' the orifices of the Heart, so that one cannot think clearly. As the Heart opens into the tongue, this consequently gives slurred and incoherent speech.

6. Stagnation of Blood in the Heart

This is very close to angina pectoris and coronary heart disease in Western medicine. It is a situation of deficiency of Heart qi giving a stagnation of Blood, which is therefore in local excess.

Symptoms are palpitations, pain around the heart that is stabbing if mild but colicky, radiating to shoulder arms, back and neck if severe. There is a feeling of fullness, stuffiness and heaviness in the chest, blueness of lips and nails, a dark purple tongue, or purple spots upon the tongue. The pulse may slow or miss beats. All these symptoms, save the palpitations, come from Blood stagnation around the Heart, leading to lack of blood in distant parts (e.g. tongue, lips and nails) and if the pain radiates down the left arm, sensations along the Heart meridian. So Blood stagnation is both the result of the disease and a causative factor obstructing the vessels. The patient experiences this as pain.

The deficient Heart syndrome that gives rise to this comes from usually either Heart yang weak or Heart Blood weak. Consequently the main underlying causes are:

(a) Mental 'irritation', i.e. emotional worries, fears, repressed anger, sadness, grief, leading to stagnation of qi. Qi guides the Blood; so stagnant qi leads to stagnant Blood. Mental irritation upsets the shen, which is based physiologically in Blood, so Heart Blood in particular stagnates.

(b) Insufficient Heart qi after a long illness or chronic ill health, so Heart is too weak to pump blood.

Summary

Deficient situations are: Heart qi; Heart yang; Heart yin; Heart Blood. However, deficient Heart qi and Heart yin usually coexist. Also, deficient Heart qi and Heart Blood often coexist; likewise, deficiency of Heart yin and yang.

Excess conditions are: Heart Fire; Derangement of the Mind. Mixed deficiency and excess occurs in Heart Blood Stagnation.

These distinctions are important; the syndromes manifest at different stages of disease. The common factor is what the Chinese call 'mental irritation', and the reason that the same causative factor leads to different syndromes is that people have different constitutions and body builds. Those with strong constitutions and body builds usually get excess syndromes, whereas the opposite applies to deficient constitutions. Consequently those who tend to be deficient in yin get deficient yin and false yang excess, whereas deficient yang types get deficient yang or deficient qi.

Apart from derangement and heart Blood stagnation, these syndromes usually appear as complications of other zangfu syndromes.

Astrologically, we have to determine within astrological constraints what strength our client has. A strong man who has been under stress for many years can take it better than a weak man who has failed to keep his qi moving. But if stress builds up, the strong man will be weakened, and if mental irritation continues he will be more likely to suffer from an excess Heart Fire situation, where fear — perhaps trifling, perhaps major — may play an important role in his life. It might be a fear of failure, or a fear of flying. The former will be more draining than the latter, which can, however, have a paralysing effect when he needs to go abroad. The strong constitution develops powerful apprehensions, superstitions and impulses; as the strain begins to show, he gets strange ideas, he blurts things out, he dislikes work, he loses his confidence. He hurries, and his co-ordination suffers. He drinks. This kind of person is materialistic, and he develops materialistic fears; but he also loses hold of his reason, becomes lonely, fears the dark, death and disease. He craves sweets, and likes open air activities that cool. He fears crowds and closed spaces. His headache feels as if it would burst and is often better for holding tight. His eyes are bloodshot and may contain pus. He gets tremors in his throat and squeamishness in his stomach. He probably smokes, and prefers cold food.

In his chart we look for a strong Jupiterian ambition with Martian need for self-enjoyment, leading to aggression. The Wood and Fire phases will predominate. We can now see how such an individual arrives at this condition. Prolonged mental stress in a strongly yang type sends energy upwards, and he shows Liver Fire and Heart Fire syndromes of red face and eyes; Wood hurries him; disturbed shen upsets his mental clarity and co-ordination, both mental and physical. He drinks and smokes to cool and calm himself (although drinking alcohol has a heating effect in the long run). Anxiety develops as his Heart and shen lose contact with Blood, and he looks with increasing desperation at external security, his job, his future, his money. His fears make him lonely and his mental state allows him fewer friends. He feels hot and dry, so likes drinking and eating cold food — if food interests him at all, as he may suffer from flatulence — another Wood phenomenon (Windy!), when Liver qi stagnates. Whatever his fears, they are quite definite — the dark, crowds, etc., and they usually relate to loss of self. Bursting headache comes from Liver fire, as do the bloodshot eyes. Throat tremors and squeamishness arise from Wood (Liver) attacking Earth (Stomach); if the attack were strong, he would feel nauseous and might vomit, in which case the vomit would be sour, derived from Wood.

Scrutiny of the chart also shows whether there is an underlying cause which makes the man chase his ambitions too hard; one of the other phases perhaps. This may require psychotherapy in addition to treatment. But it has to be said that such excess yang types turn with reluctance to unorthodox medicine, which may undermine their self-confidence at first. If they turn to it, they do so with embarrassment and may avoid telling associates, who might think they were mad!

Path of Fire Phase Channels

The Heart meridian originates in the heart, spreads over the surrounding area, sending one branch down to the small intestine. Another branch ascends beside the oesophagus up to the eyes. The main meridian goes to the lung, and emerges in the axilla, from where it travels along the posterior medial aspect of the arm to the palm and small finger.

The Small Intestine meridian starts from the small finger and follows the ulnar edge of the hand and arm to the elbow, then to the shoulder, posterior aspect. It circles the scapula, reaches across to the seventh cervical vertebra, from which a branch connects with the heart, through the diaphragm to the stomach and small intestine. From the shoulder it ascends to the neck, jaw and cheek, entering the ear and eyes.

The Pericardium channel originates in the chest and enters the pericardium sending a branch down through the abdomen connecting upper, middle and lower jiao. The main branch emerges close to the axilla and runs down the medial aspect of the arm to elbow, and on to wrist, palm and middle finger. A branch goes from palm to the ring finger, where it becomes the Three Heater channel.

The Three Heater channel starts on the tip of the ring finger, runs between fourth and fifth metacarpal bones to dorsal aspect of the wrist and lateral aspect of the arm, through posterior elbow and up the lateral aspect of the upper arm to the shoulder. It goes over the supraclavicular fossa to the neck, up behind and round the ear to the cheek below the eye. A branch enters the ear; emerging, it crosses the cheek to the outer canthus of the eye, linking there with the Gall Bladder channel.

Fire types may or may not experience pain along these channels, but they often experience stomach upsets and, *in extremis*, pain in chest, neck and arm as described.

Case 4. Female, 76

Chart 4 gives a typical case of heart problems. The patient was 76, had been a hairdresser for many years and had then sold flowers in a very cold shop. Her presenting complaint was pain, described as of osteoarthritic origin by her doctor, up the outside of her left leg from ankle to hip. In fact she had pulled a calf muscle some six months earlier when swimming, and had been on pain-killing drugs for the ensuing period. The pain was excruciating, and the pain-killers had little effect; it gnawed and throbbed like a knife being pushed in and turned.

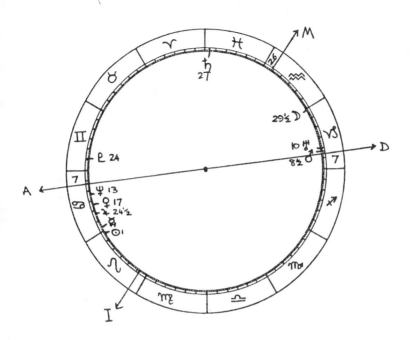

Chart 4. Female, 76.

Three years ago her back gave way and X-rays showed worn discs, which the use of a walking-stick had helped, and she reported that this was now all right. Eight years ago she had had high blood pressure and was given tablets, and said that she used to get palpitations and headaches: her doctor had diagnosed angina. She had varicose veins badly on both legs.

Her sleep, she said, was very erratic — with luck three hours per night, and she could only sleep on her right, a side she had never slept on before. She had many dreams, like visions, and frequently they foretold the future. Appetite was good, which was a pity (she gaily remarked!) as she was very obese — hence the anti-obesity drugs she was also taking. She disliked alcohol but took lots of coffee, which she liked, and fruit juice. She had never smoked. She was red-faced, laughed a lot and was great fun.

She was diagnosed as having excess Heart Fire, deficient Heart qi and a dysfunction along the Gall Bladder meridian line. Her blood pressure was 190/90, but her heartbeat was normal. She was not usually very thirsty. She had had three children and one miscarriage.

Her presenting complaint of leg pain was the least of her problems, but it was the one which modern medicine had failed to eradicate. The other problems Western medicine was controlling to some extent. Her chart is that of someone with plenty of energy, who had difficulty in controlling her tendency to overactivity (♂ ☌ ♅ ☍ A; ☉ ☍ ☽: planets in 1st house). She admitted that she had always pushed herself too hard, but at 76 she still had the enthusiasm for life of a 30-year-old. Her problems were clearly those of a very active woman, and the pain intensity was one of excess, as were the red face and the general exuberance. Interestingly she came when T♄$_{♏}$ ☌ P (☿ + ☽) △A$_{♋}$ although the angina had occurred when P☉ ☌ T♇ □A, P☽ ☌ ☉$_{R}$, P♂ ☍ ♃$_{R}$.

In such a chart we expect Wood and Fire problems: with ♆ ☌ A we may also expect poor restraint on yin (see ♆, later), and indeed she was obese. The interesting matter is that treatment was directed not at the pain, but at the overactivity of Heart, and at controlling yin. Although 76, she could be expected to respond very well, and after the first treatment she said that she had slept better than before pulling her calf muscle; she could now drop off at any time and wake refreshed; the leg pain was also gone. In fact she felt so much better that she had overdone things again and her back was hurting, though she was inclined to leave her stick behind. In spite of a large family gathering at Christmas she had not felt particularly hungry, save at meals. After some large meals she still got headaches and flushes, so was continuing with the angina pills. She had one further treatment (two in all) and was advised that she ought to have longer treatment to deal with the underlying problem (i.e. Heart).

However, no more was heard until several months later when her daughter called to say that her mother's leg had been much better and also her sleep. Unfortunately she had recently overeaten again, and had caught a 'gall bladder infection', which had given her chest pains, and so she had been rushed to hospital with a suspected heart attack. The hospital wanted to remove the gall bladder, but insisted that she lose weight first, so she was now at home, her general cheerfulness only slightly marred by the fact that she was on a starvation diet!

4.

VENUS ♀

Venus has always been associated with value and with beauty and the fairest of the species — to be admired. If Mars is our ability for cheerful self-assertion and self-enjoyment, Venus represents our desire to be improved, given quality, essence, life, by that which self-asserts. So it is not so much our desire to relate as our need to let ourselves *be* related to. This depends to some extent on the value we put upon ourselves, and the feeling of well-being we derive from our background and from our love of ourselves. The Venus area of the chart shows in which walk of life we find contentment in being valued. For easy reciprocal relationships it should preferably not be too close to the Ascendant, nor placed in a backward-looking or introverted area such as the 4th house, though if here placed it could suggest a happy married life and a pleasant home environment, but no special need for very outgoing relationships.

But if the ability to be related to depends on our sense of well-being, then Venus also shows how easily we exchange energy, how we colour it with our feelings. From another person's point of view it represents in us our contribution in terms of quality of life and of personality, but not the energy with which we give ourselves to our fellows, which comes from the more yang planets like the Sun, Mars and Jupiter.

Venus placed powerfully in a chart gives its possessor a special area of class, of beauty, of desirability. These people bring to their relationships an intensely personal and intimate touch, and those who come within their orbit feel honoured and at times almost bewitched. Such people operate best when we seek them out; they are less happy when they have to make the running themselves! This points to an underlying laziness — from our point of view. But why should they seek us when they feel so good with themselves — when they can attract others just by being what they are. They have the powerful ability to share themselves with us, and we, each of us, want to feel ennobled by them. This is their strength.

But strength needs to be recognized, and a rich miser cuts himself off from life if he hides his wealth. What use is light, if kept hidden? The rich man — or he who aims to become rich — must learn the true value of riches. He must sell his labours for a fair deal, he must be willing to use his capital if he wants to grow richer, and he must reinvigorate his community with the fruits of his success. Art treasures should be shared to be enjoyed. Knowledge gained must be taught. That which has been received must be returned, or how can it be valued? In the process of returning what we have received, we enrich it with our own essence, thereby invigorating life as a whole.

This idea of value received and quality given accords with the energy of Metal. The Metal phase lies between the happy, outgoing self-assertiveness of Fire, and the quiet, waiting and adjusting, absorbing phase of Water. Fire throws its energy forward; Metal is the receiver of that thrust. It separates the ash from the fire, sending it down into the earth, and uses the volatile gas given off by the flames as energy, 'qi'. These two aspects of fire, vapour and ash, are all that remains when Fire burns low; yet they are what must carry on the cycle of life. Their importance is just as great as that of any other phase. They are the weight of experience, the judgement refined from years of ardour, the wisdom of balance. No wonder we all want that balance! We want to seem wise, experienced, knowledgeable, at peace with ourselves, sought out, desirable, something special! — and perhaps these are qualities we display when the Metal phase flows smoothly.

Unfortunately you don't notice it when Metal is working well. (As Zen enlightenment dawned, a man called it 'grey', although he didn't mean dull.) In practice we notice Metal when the phase gets blocked, and there is no longer that ready exchange of energy and ash; instead we feel stuffed up and undesirable; or we rush around searching desperately for the secret of life, berating ourselves or our parents for being unworthy, useless, discarded or unnecessary. We are certainly not nice to know, yet we try ever so hard to be nice and cultivated. We feel ourselves to be boring; so, fearing that we bore others, we avoid relationships that expand us. Yet rush we must or accept the dullness of our lives.

Metal phase imbalance types are supposed to show grief, the emotion associated with Metal; but grief for the loss of another, if it remains too long, is more likely to be a stuck Liver syndrome. Metal grief is grief and despair for ourselves, and we hide it, or refuse to

admit it. Once we can admit it, and let go of it, and no doubt cry
our hearts out while doing so, we can then readjust and move on,
healthy at least in Metal.

The laugh of Metal is not the warm laugh of a loving Fire, or the
exuberant laugh of an ambitious Wood, but an understanding,
accepting smile of shared experience.

More than anything else we share air, the least substantial necessity
of life, without which we die in a few minutes. The lungs are the
yin organs of Metal. The other things we share are our faeces, our
sweat and — when it finally flakes off — our skin. As the man said,
'Life is like a drainpipe; what you get out of it depends on what you
put in!' So the other Metal-associated functional systems are the Large
Intestine and the skin, which in this system of Medicine comes under
Venus, the planet of exchange, contact and value. But if we imagine
someone who breathes deeply and naturally, whose intestines
regularly jettison what is not needed, whose skin has lustre and tone,
whose voice has power and depth, and contrast this with a patient
who has a cold, is constipated and stuffed up, with no energy and
a miserable outlook, we can see how Metal affects us. Mentally, good
breathing gives us a calm certainty and self-possession; physically
it relaxes us and rhythmically it massages the contents of our
abdomen. Like all the yin planets, Venus has a relation to rhythm
and natural repeated actions that constitute the role of nourishment.

Functions of the Lungs

1. Lungs govern respiration

Harmonious, rhythmic breathing exhales stale air and disperses pure
new qi about the organism, so the thorax is called the 'reservoir of
qi'. The action of the lungs is calming. A few deep breaths in a tense
situation help to relax us and to clear our minds, so the lungs are
said to send energies downwards. If the Lungs work properly, all
energies in the body will be in good order.

When they lose their function of dominating breathing and
dispersing qi properly, we suffer from shallow breathing and a weak
voice. If Lung qi gets stuck we get a full, stuffy chest with coughing
and difficulty in breathing. If Lungs fail to send energy down, we
may suffer from a puffy face and skin, phlegm in our sinuses, nasal
discharge, dyspnoea and difficulty in catching our breath.

2. Lungs dominate qi

We take in the energy of 'Heaven' through our noses and absorb
it in our lungs. The Lungs connect us directly to the source of all

energy outside us, and it is within the Lungs that the qi absorbed from food mixes with the qi from Heaven to form useful qi for our bodies.

Consequently the quality of Lung qi determines the quality of qi throughout the entire organism; and the function of the Lungs determines how it is distributed rhythmically around the body.

(Astrological note: Venus is the planet of co-operation and partnership; here we see how it is the source of the quality of life.)

'Heavenly' or 'Cosmic' qi is hard to appreciate, but we may grasp what is meant by leaving a city full of smoke and fumes and going up a nearby mountain to breathe the air, look at the view and feel refreshed and exhilarated in spirit, mind and body. It gives a feeling of order and pattern which may be hidden from us when below. This energy is infinitely abundant; through our bodies we refine it and make our lives. It also regulates the strength of the organism, not in terms of muscular strength but in our ability to meet adversity and remain healthy and integrated, to face disease and attack, and to cohere.

When this qi is insufficient we have low vitality, fatigue, low spirits, lethargy and melancholy. If we have too much, we become hyper-ventilated, with giddiness, drunkenness and hysterical over-exuberance.

3. Lung qi leads the Blood and its pulse

There is some overlap here with the functions of the Heart, which controls the Blood and pulse. But there is a subtle distinction. In traditional Chinese medicine, the relationship between qi and Blood is an aspect of that between yang and yin, and whole volumes have been devoted to it. In this book it is discussed in Chapter 8. For present purposes, their interdependence may be summarized by saying that 'qi is the leader of the Blood, but Blood is the attachment of qi'. So Blood and qi travel together, as Heart is master of Blood, and Lungs are master of qi. (In addition, Heart yang moves qi.)

If Lungs are weak, we may be anaemic and have poor circulation; our pulse might be slow or intermittent; or there might be palpitation as Heart yang desperately tries to compensate for deficient qi. (Another traditional name for Lungs is 'little Heart'.)

As one would expect, it is the qi of the Lungs which is said to initiate a new meridian energy cycle every day at 3 a.m. as the yang of the day begins to manifest. Illness at this time can point to Lung weakness.

It is worth emphasizing that the only cells where the energy o the Lungs fails to penetrate are dead cells. An abundance of good Lung qi is a strong safeguard against any form of cancer, where the cells seem able to live on lower levels of qi, and for healthy regulation of diseased or traumatized tissues. 'Qigong' is a discipline out of which Tai Qi has arisen; it teaches the facility to be so focussed that qi is actually directed through the body by mental concentration and appropriate breathing. In the West some of the mental visualization exercises developed to help cancer sufferers are a move in this direction. In traditional Chinese medicine there are several reasons for cancer; an important one is stagnation of Blood. As we have seen, stagnation can occur, for instance, when Liver is stuck, but there is another cause: Lung qi failing to lead the Blood. The opposite is also true: any stagnation of Blood leads to deterioration in Lung qi.

4. Lungs move and regulate the water channels

Water metabolism is an important function of the Lungs, which have a direct relation to the Kidneys in traditional Chinese medicine. Part of their dispersive function is to turn body fluids into sweat to be excreted through the skin. The Lungs themselves need moisture which they receive from the Kidney yang, and without which there is dryness in breathing and coughing, dry skin, dry nose and throat. The Lungs have a paired organ, the Large Intestine, whose actions they also dominate. The Large Intestine assimilates water from the faeces. (The Lungs receive what is called Impure fluid from Spleen yang and send it to Kidney yin. If they fail we see facial oedema and puffiness, and Kidney inflammation.)

5. Lungs rule energy of skin and body hair

(Hair on the head is ruled mainly by Kidney energy.)

The skin is our third lung, and the Lungs send moisture to nourish it and give it lustre. The skin is the outside surface of the body and its tone comes from Lung qi. It is our first line of defence, and defensive (Wei) qi is directed by Lung qi, so Lungs protect us on the outside. The great enemy of the Lungs is Dryness. If weak, they may also be unable to summon enough Wei qi, so we get a cold skin, catch cold easily, and sweat without exertion. Lung qi is responsible through Wei qi for opening and closing the pores of the skin, and many a cold has been caught, according to traditional Chinese medicine, by people whose pores remain open too long for sweating after exercise, and have allowed cold and wind ingress. The moral is: when sweating from exercise, keep well wrapped up; cool down a bit while so covered, then undress quickly and shower, finishing off with a quick cool shower. In this way we do not allow ourselves to cool down too fast, leaving our pores open to 'catch a chill'. If undressing is unavoidable after heavy perspiration, avoid draughts and breathe calmly and deeply.

Those who find they perspire even when unheated or when not taking exercise — i.e. spontaneous sweating during the day — may be suffering from weak Lungs and/or weak Wei qi.

6. Lungs open into the nose and throat
This gives us a good sense of smell, easy breathing and a good timbre to the voice. The voice carries the quality of the qi of the organism, so can be a diagnostic factor in disease. Throat problems caused by dryness or mucus are often due to Lung or Stomach deficiency; those caused by swellings (e.g. of the lymph nodes) are more likely to be due to Stomach or Large Intestine.

7. Sorrow, anxiety, melancholy, worry
Too much of these emotions may damage the Lungs, or be a sign of their malfunction. Each involves a continual holding on to something, either in the past or in the future. The right lung is affected by grief and sadness, which disperse the whole energy of the body. The left lung is more affected by worry, which is said to coagulate the qi. Melancholy and over-thinking are also associated with Spleen problems, but melancholy in particular also affects the Lungs.

8. Lungs and instincts
There are several Chinese descriptions of what we might call instinct. Relevant to the lungs is *p'o*, which we might equate with hereditary instincts and programming, our instinctual impulse. When we become obsessed with this, we become obsessed with the future, and apprehensive about it. If deficient, we lack the instinct for self-preservation, so may be vulnerable and lack aggression, perhaps weeping at our uselessness. We lack the wherewithal to deal with stress. We are open to it and need to learn to defend ourselves.

9. Lung associations (See also Appendix)
The associations most useful are those of sound and smell. If Lung energy is imbalanced, the primary sound made when talking is one of crying — not shouting, but plaintive and sorry for itself. The smell is like rotten meat or fish.

Dry weather in excess injures lungs and skin, and is the source of some lung problems. In China, in the central area, autumn is an extremely hot, dry period, when diseases associated with the lungs are more likely to begin.

Sense organ: the nose.

Syndromes of the Lung

Syndromes of the Lung are not restricted to the lungs, but extend to the whole respiratory system, including for example throat and nose. When the Lung is diseased, symptoms often appear in these areas. Because Lungs are part of Metal phase, there is often a corresponding energy imbalance in Large Intestine, the other Metal phase energy, and in its associated organ, the Colon. However, such symptoms may also be treated via the energy of the Stomach or Spleen meridians, which are the originators of phlegm that is said to be stored in the Lung. There is therefore a close relationship between the Earth and the Metal phase energy, and some Metal phase problems are due to problems which stem from Earth.

1. Invasion of Lungs by external Wind Heat;
2. Invasion of Lungs by external Wind Cold;
3. Phlegm Damp in the Lungs;
4. Phlegm Heat in the Lungs;
5. Deficient Lung yin;
6. Deficient Lung qi.

(In one sense, deficient qi of the Lungs (6) may be responsible for all the others save deficient Lung yin. If there is sufficient qi, then external influences cannot invade, nor can phlegm collect.)

1. Invasion by external Wind
This is often seen in the 'common cold', bronchitis, etc.

2a. Invasion by external Wind Heat
External Heat signs include: a fever that is more prominent than chilliness (there may even be no sense of chilliness); aches over the body are more intense than with Wind Cold; there is more tension, the pain tearing or burning or tingling; heaviness, but there is external soreness too; perspiration, dark yellow urine, constipation (faeces are dried out), tongue is red, its covering is yellow, and any expectoration is sticky and yellow, even green. Attack on the Lungs shows up with nasal obstruction and a yellow, purulent discharge; throat is red, dry, burning and constricted, with difficulty in swallowing; there may be a cough, which is dry and hoarse, with

shortness of breath, and somewhat worse for drinking, especially hot liquids. If the heat dries the liquids, then the nose will be dry and may bleed, and will be acutely sensitive to smells; and in this case any discharge will be hot, scanty and watery. Notice that although there are many signs of heat and dryness, there is often difficulty drinking because of the constriction, and because the heat has not dried out internal fluids, there is usually no thirst.

It is interesting to understand why these acute conditions come about. Invasion of skin and hair by External Wind gives rise to chilliness and fever; the Wind causes the sensations to move around the body, hence the restlessness. Invasion of the throat and mouth by Wind affects the lungs, causing cough, sputum, sore throat, nasal obstruction and runny nose, etc.

In considering how to treat these different forms of Wind invasion, e.g. common cold, bronchitis, tonsillitis, bronchial asthma etc., we must first differentiate between Wind Cold and Wind Heat. On a practical level, the Wind Cold patient lacks yang to combat the disease; he should be kept warm and be given warming foods and liquids. The Wind Heat type may be better for open air and cooling liquids, if he can swallow them; he is also usually better for gentle exercise and an upright posture, whereas the Cold type is better for lying down and a warm bed.

2b. Invasion by external Wind Cold

Signs of external Cold invasion include: chilliness, possibly with a mild fever (the chilliness is more prominent, and there is sometimes no fever); aching all over the body, which may feel heavy or bruised; a dull pain up and down the spine; lack of perspiration; light-coloured urine and perhaps loose stools.

Signs of Lung imbalance include itching in the throat, a loud cough, nasal obstruction, a clear runny discharge from the nose, and sputum that is white and dilute. The tongue has a thin white covering, and there may be difficulty breathing: there is often a headache.

3. Retention of Phlegm Damp Cold in Lung

The situation has now moved from an exterior syndrome to an interior syndrome: Lung deficiency has now allowed phlegm to build up, a sign of excess. Consequently there are no external signs of Cold, at least in a pure form of the syndrome. However, attack of the syndrome is often exacerbated by cold weather. Symptoms are mainly respiratory, including cough, an oppressed heavy feeling in the chest, difficulty breathing (which is better sitting up) and expectoration of copious thick, white, frothy sputum. Tongue covering is white and can be sticky. The more Phlegm Damp exists, the thicker and stickier is the sputum. Here the main cause is weak Spleen, but Lungs act as 'container of the sputum'. As the cause is a weak Spleen, there is often nausea and vomiting.

4. Retention of Phlegm Heat in Lungs

This is an interior, excess type of syndrome, often seen in febrile diseases caused by invasion of external pathogenic factors. Whereas Phlegm Damp Cold is usually long-lasting and slow to resolve, Phlegm Heat is severe, acute and can be dangerous. Symptoms are cough, asthmatic breathing, much thick, purulent yellow or green sputum, which because of the Heat may be bloody, and smell foul. There is usually a fever. Here the patient feels better in the open air. The tongue is red with a yellow covering. The patient may look flushed. The cough is worse for eating, better for cool air. There may be itchiness or dryness of the skin. As the Heat burns deeper, there is profuse easy sweating and the urine is dark and may burn. This picture is close to that of empyema, following on from pneumonia. Usually there is mental anxiety, if not agitation.

5. Deficient yin of Lung

Deficiency of yin leads to relative excess of yang of Lung; so as well as general signs of yin deficiency we expect signs of weak Heat in the Lung. Signs of yin deficiency include dryness of skin and mouth, red cheeks, and even a feeling of heat especially in the afternoon, a thin, perhaps emaciated body, spontaneous perspiration at night, a tongue that is red, the pulse a little fast. Lung yin signs are a dry cough, worse after noon; desire for fresh, cool but not cold air; very little phlegm; blood coughed up, laryngitis and hoarseness. He is generally worse from 3 a.m. to 6 a.m. and at night, worse for cold air and cold drinks, better for cool flannels on the forehead, and better lying down, though the restlessness often prevents this. Notice that the more qi there is, the less desired will be rest. The great craving will be for cold open air, cold drinks and gentle motion.

This patient's energy is sporadic; he easily tires, but after a rest rallies and has great schemes and emotional outbursts. He is often highly irritable. Because the p'o is affected, the instinctual drives are disordered, and the desire for change is strong. Sexual energy is weak but the patient is willing, then exhausted. The patient has great ups and downs!

This syndrome is usually caused either by an invasion of external

Wind Heat or a deficiency of Kidney yin.

6. Deficient qi of Lungs

The Lungs dominate qi, so weak Lung qi also gives signs of weak qi. There is a look of tiredness and exhaustion, a weak voice, weak breathing, spontaneous sweating, dislike of talking, a white face; often feels the cold, and catches cold easily; any coughing is weak. The pulse is weak, the tongue pale. As there is weak qi and this is the Metal phase, we might expect also to find constipation without urging; no power to strain, even if the faeces are soft. There may be hair loss.

This condition arises from a chronic lung disease, e.g. cough, which has weakened the Lungs; or from an internal problem such as a long period of worry or grief, allied perhaps to overwork. It can also be caused by weak qi of Heart and Spleen. The patient loses his normal instincts and his reflexes are slow.

Route of Metal Phase Meridians

The Lung Channel originates in the middle chou, from which it sends a branch to the large intestine. It ascends through the upper orifice of the stomach, through the diaphragm and enters the lungs, from which it contacts the throat, then passes to a point just inferior to the distal extremity of the clavicle. It proceeds along the medial aspect of the arm, through the elbow and continues to the wrist, where it enters the radial artery, ending at the thumb. From the wrist it sends a branch to the tip of the index finger, from which point the Large Intestine Channel begins.

The Large Intestine Channel passes through the web of flesh between thumb and first finger, along the lateral aspect of the forearm to the lateral angle of the elbow crease, up the arm to the top of the shoulder, from which it passes to the seventh cervical vertebra, to the supraclavicular fossa, to lungs, diaphragm and large intestine. A branch from the supraclavicular fossa ascends the neck through the sternocleidomastoideus muscle to the cheek, gums of lower jaw, crossing above the upper lip to the opposite side of the nose.

Venus in Western astrology is traditionally associated with the lower back and kidneys, the throat, circulation especially the veins. More recently it has been associated with the parathyroid glands.

Traditional Chinese medicine gives the Lungs domination over the qi, so we can widen Venus's rulership to include arterial circulation. In Western astrology its connection with the lower back and kidneys is well known, and we shall be in a better position to study this when we have considered the Water phase. However, if the Lungs fail to send energy down to the Kidneys, then we shall make greater inroads on Kidney qi, and this may lead to a sore back (amongst other things). We have to remember that without qi, there is no movement and no warmth, so Lung deficiency will lead to many kinds of circulatory problems, including arthritis.

In traditional Chinese medicine the Lungs play an important part in the Water cycle of the body, and they are responsible for some aspects of excretion.

Venus's relationship with the throat and, via Taurus, with singers is clearer when we see how important is the role of the Lungs in producing a smooth and powerful voice; and when we consider the paths of the Metal phase meridians through the throat. (Other meridians also pass up the neck, but the majority of throat problems due to invasion by external pathogenic forces are treated clinically mainly on the Large Intestine and the Lung channels.)

5.

MERCURY ☿

The greatest contribution traditional Chinese medicine has to make to Western astrology is in its understanding of Kidney energy, and of the importance of Mercury in the chart.

In Western astrology, Mercury is often ignored or treated as being unimportant compared with the Sun, with which it frequently forms conjunctions. There is a message here: Mercury and the Sun are aspects of the same energy, and are closer than any other two energies. The Heart (Mars), and Lungs (Venus) are in the upper chou. The Kidneys (Mercury) are in the lower chou. All three are personal planets — they have a direct relationship to the way we express ourselves, yet Mercury is often so close to the Sun that it is hard to distinguish its meaning.

Western astrology says that Mercury shows the ability to communicate and to co-ordinate ideas. This process is achieved through the conscious thinking processes and through the senses of the nervous system, all of which are ruled by Mercury. Mercury shows the need to communicate and learn, the urge to know and to be conscious. This requires an ability to adapt oneself to the learning environment, and to look for variety and change, so that one can manipulate the environment to one's own advantage. It therefore comes close to being one's intellect: well placed, it gives a round grasp of ideas with good critical ability and mental dexterity, useful both manipulatively and diplomatically. Poorly placed it gives inability to understand, to remember, and wastefulness of mental energy in too many directions, with difficulty communicating. Poorly placed it can sometimes point to a genius that burns itself out, lacking persistence and consistency.

Mercury is related to the Water phase; this is the quiescent phase of night, rest, winter. How can we reconcile this with Mercury's adaptability, avoidance of routine and need to learn?

Mercury is the planet closest to the Sun (with the possible exception of another planet, its discovery long awaited, Vulcan, said to rule Virgo). Symbolically one may call it the first precipitation of the energy of life into material reality. It may therefore be both the foundation for all other planetary energies, and contain within it the greatest amount of raw energy, forever releasing kinetically. Mercury has more frequent changes of direction (retrograde motion) as seen from Earth than any other planet. Its direction may be forward but it often goes backward, another sign of its seeking release of energy in all possible ways, of its duality. If we over-use our Mercury energy it quickly runs down although, being so close to the Sun, it recovers fast. So it has terrific potential, and it is to the credit of the genius of the ancient Chinese that they associated the planet of greatest duality, liveliness and vigour with the phase of greatest potential energy.

For the Kidney energy does not move and expand like Jupiter, or express itself like Mars, or give quality and refinement of experience, like Venus: nor is it the base through which the rest function, like Saturn. It contains within itself the balancing power of yin and yang, on which all the other energies rely to a greater or lesser extent. Its yin function is to balance the outgoing energy of Jupiter and Mars; its yang function is to be the pilot light for the energy needed to digest and refine what is absorbed through Saturn and Venus. Whereas Saturn provides the ground of a physical body, Mercury provides a stabilizing influence; it enables us to adapt ourselves back to a position of harmony from either one of action and movement, or one of absorption and reflection.

The modern world requires more adaptability and learning than did that of the ancients; we have to think and move faster to stay alive. Except in the countryside, we have largely lost touch with the healing process of the seasons, although religious and traditional festivals try to maintain an awareness of the yearly cycle. In ancient times, winter meant less light, a natural restriction we can now ignore. It was therefore a period of greater rest, more gathering round the community fires, greater time to reflect and to meditate and to learn to be patient. It was a time to eat stores, to restrain activity and to keep warm. So man conserved his store of essential qi, often perforce. Today's city-dwellers need observe no such rituals: winter is when — having overworked — we rush home in the evening and then head for adult evening classes; when we eat and drink more, rather than less, the parties in our heated homes searching out the small hours. We can submit to our need for change and our horror of boredom by holidaying abroad, often strenuously up mountains, or overheated by an overhead sun. And when we get bored with that, we have computers to play with and drugs to suppress our fears, anxieties, tensions, insomnias and regrets — not to mention our peptic ulcers! We have other medicines to revitalize us from our depression and lift us from our sorrow.

All of these we need because we have ignored and forgotten the essential balancing function of our Water phase energy, the Kidney qi, yin, yang and jing (see below) ruled by the planet Mercury.

Mercury is a two-sided planet, more adaptable than any other. The process of communication has two sides, absorption and transmission: movement and rest are relative. More than any other planet, it is able to represent the duality of Kidney energy; and more than any other the Kidney has duality, a yin and yang side that form the basis of all yin and yang in the body, but which are not *the* yin (=Blood) or *the* yang (=qi) of the body. Mercury similarly contains the germ of the other planets; without its fluidity there can be no change, no nutrition and no absorption. To those planets that give expansion and warmth and change, it acts as a memory which anchors them in reality. For planets that give stability and balance it gives the contrast of purpose and vitality. Each finds its balance within Mercury.

The Water phase is at the end of one cycle, and the start of the next. It is a natural pause, when the seed that was sown lies dormant. We end one cycle by ploughing into the land all the old rubbish. And there it sits, a graveyard. Old buildings lose their owners and decay, eventually becoming archaeological sites, or ploughed up into new fields. Garbage dumps contain rich food for the future. But it takes a pause before we realize what riches lie buried in our past. If we force new growth from the field or the plant before it has had time to rest, it will outgrow its strength and we shall be unable to repeat the process. For those who believe in reincarnation, the period between lives is an unknown; but the new body learns the essential ingredients to continue the chain, and the gap represents a sifting process, when the life that is to be is said to perceive its identity, uncluttered by memories of the past; its memory is simply a realization of who it is, and what its purpose is to be. So Mercury can be seen as the seed from the past, the encapsulated genetic survival code, awaiting new experience.

The hours of sleep are the same, and we should awaken with renewed energy if our Liver has functioned properly. But the Liver has its roots in Kidney yin, as Jupiter has its roots in Mercury, and it is Mercury that knows the way to and from the depths: Mercury — Hermes — God of travellers, and protector of flocks; he opens and closes the gate on this retreat where we go to concentrate our energies anew.

Functions of the Kidneys

1. Kidneys store jing

Jing can be translated as 'essence'; this is a substance that comes out of the bond between our parents and which becomes the foundation of our native, inborn constitution. Sensible food, properly eaten, can to some extent replenish it. Jing governs reproduction, growth and development throughout life; when it runs out, we die; consequently old people — and, increasingly, young people who have abused themselves — show symptoms of Kidney jing deficiency. Jing determines the constitution of the next generation. If sufficient jing exists, a child's growth will be normal, with bones, teeth and hair appearing at appropriate intervals, the brain developing and puberty coming on naturally. Infertility, impotence and menopausal problems can be due to jing deficiency.

Besides governing our natural growth processes, jing provides a reservoir of life essence in times of trauma, such as shock, accidents, bad news, prolonged over-exertion and haemorrhage. Using up too many seminal fluids (sperm or vaginal) has the effect of draining jing.

It is said to govern in women a seven-year cycle of life, in men an eight-year cycle. On this basis, women at 14 have their menarche, and men at 16 their puberty; at 28 (women) and 32 (men), Kidney qi is at its zenith, the prime of life. At 49 (women) and 64 (men) Kidney qi begins to decline and the reproductive ability fails. Modern experience is that these ages are, in at least the case of puberty, too high.

Kidney jing is an aspect of Kidney yin, because it is deemed to be a fluid. Kidney yang is the active function of the Kidney; and in order that life may proceed, there must be qi, in the same way that life as we know it is impossible in the interstellar gaseous fluid (yin) unless the fluids of space coalesce into matter and are heated in such a way that life may evolve, life being qi and Blood. Jing is an underlying force of nature, such as gravity, that brings the situation to fruition. These underlying forces are a property of the nature of matter (yin) itself; they hold together in times of stress and, if they fail, we crack up and eventually die.

The relationship of jing to the brain becomes clearer seen in this light. The Chinese did not see the mind and the brain quite as we see them, and we must ask what part of ourselves holds us together when all our other defences have failed. The answer may be our individual appreciation of the function and strength of Kidney jing. Equally it equates with our vitality for life. Jing is vitally important in the creation of our spinal cord and brain, and in the formation of the blood-forming marrow of our bones. Many deep-rooted fears about life are treated via the Kidney, as are many diseases associated with the brain, such as meningitis and some forms of paralysis. Equally, as we shall see, one cause of weakness of intellect and dizziness is deficiency of Kidney jing.

2. Kidneys produce 'marrow', control bones, fill brain, make Blood

'Marrow' is a misleading term and needs to be understood. It is not bone marrow or bone, but the energy idea behind them. The brain and spinal cord are in traditional Chinese medicine called the 'Sea of Marrow', yet the substance of the brain is not 'bone marrow'. If this 'Sea of Marrow' is well-nourished by Kidney jing, we develop clear cogent powers of thought, perception and memory; if not, our minds are confused and dull, we get dizzy, we cannot remember, we cannot sleep and we cannot perceive what our senses tell us; for instance, our vision suffers. (There are, of course, other causes of these problems.)

Good solid bones that resist disease and contain healthy bone marrow and grow properly, and a strong back, suggest healthy Kidney jing and 'marrow'.

From this we can see how the Kidneys dominate the basic physical foundation of the body.

3. Kidneys dominate water metabolism

This domination is an active function, hence comes mainly under Kidney yang, whose job in this respect is to disperse water it receives either to the Bladder for excretion or in the form of 'vapour' to those organs that require it; notably it moistens the Lungs. It receives fluids from various sources; from the intestines, where it separates fluid from solid; from the Lungs, which send down fluids that are a mixture of clear and turbid. It controls with Spleen yang the dispersion of water that would otherwise collect and cause oedema, such as under the eyes or in the legs and ankles. It controls urination.

4. Kidneys control reception of qi and hold it down

As the root and foundation of qi, the Kidneys attract it down to themselves.

Respiration is dominated by the Lungs, but part of the process is assisted by the Kidneys, notably inhalation. Inability to catch one's breath can be a Kidney problem.

More important is the qi inspired which the Lungs send down to the Kidneys. If the Lungs fail to 'descend' this qi, or the Kidneys fail to hold it, then the air passages get blocked and qi remains in the upper chou, causing congestion and difficulty in breathing, often diagnosed in Western medicine as asthma.

All energies require an anchor, otherwise they disperse. Being yang, qi tends to flow upwards. The Kidneys provide this anchor, and impairment of their function allows energy to float up the body, causing pain, heat and tension in upper parts and deficiency of qi and yang, e.g. coldness and stagnation, in lower parts. For example, the Liver-Kidney connection keeps Liver yang smooth. If Kidney yin fails to supply Liver yin, the Liver yang rises up, causing symptoms such as cramps and numbness, headaches, noises in the ears, irritability and insomnia.

If the Kidney-Heart relationship is impaired by deficient Kidney yin then we get palpitations, difficulty getting to sleep, dry mouth, red cheeks, dizziness, restlessness, anxiety and other mental problems.

5. Kidneys open into the ear

Although all the energies of the body are required for efficient hearing, the Kidneys are said to have particular influence on the ears. As Kidney energy decreases with age, hearing becomes less lively; tinnitus and deafness develop.

6. Kidneys control the two yin: Anus and Urethra

Kidney weakness leads to such problems as inability to complete urination and uncontrollable diarrhoea, especially in the morning.

7. Kidneys associate with fear

This fear is deep, a fear of life, a deep anxiety about one's ability to survive. It is often irrational, unfounded and unspecific. It may go back to very early life, subconscious fears, paranoia and feelings of persecution. Excess fear of any kind can injure the Kidneys; but the fear that arises from them is not easily spoken of. It is often worse at night, or in the dark. Children who cannot sleep without a light nearby may be nurturing a life-long fear of life: they need comfort and reassurance.

8. Kidneys relate to the uterus

The uterus is one of the six extra fu, but its properties are so close to those of the Kidney that the Kidneys may be said to control it to a large extent. The uterus lies in the lower chou, the area where we dump all our rubbish and excrement before excretion. The lower chou contains the anus and the urethra, source of many 'unpleasant' associations, not to mention the bad smells! Like in a pond, the mud at the bottom is very mucky stuff. But it also nurtures life, because that mud is very rich in nutrients. The female body contains this wonderful space called her 'uterus' which more than anything gives her yin essence, the ground in which creation can take place when an ovum and a sperm form a new conjunction. So the uterus, nourished by all the rich blood, dominates the menstrual cycle and pregnancy. If the Kidney energy is healthy, then the blood is likely to be good, and the mother's ability to mother will be strong: her body will know 'how'. (Of course there are other important energies associated with menstruation. The Kidneys are only one factor.)

9. General associations

Deep, biting *cold*; salty taste; fear — all, in excess, harm Kidney. The smell associated with Kidney is that of decay or putrefaction; putrid. The behaviour associated with deficient Kidney is trembling or quivering. The hair on the head is an outward manifestation of Kidney.

Two areas of the body are particularly related to Kidney: low back and knees. Strong teeth are a sign of good Kidney.

Kidney Pathology

In other organs, deficiency of Blood and qi progresses to deficiency of yin and yang as a rule. Thus, for example, qi deficiency eventually develops into yang deficiency. The Kidney situation is slightly different because they form the basis of yin and yang in the body. The expression 'Kidney qi' is loose terminology for the functional combination of Kidney yin and yang. Because the Kidneys form the basis of yin and yang, which form the basis of Blood and qi, Kidney energy is almost never in excess, but clinically it is frequently in deficiency. As mentioned earlier, Kidney jing is received at birth, and replenished only very slowly, if at all, thereafter. (But it can be kept in good order by a suitable lifestyle.) So Kidney problems are often deep, chronic and difficult to treat, and may have been inherited.

If the Kidneys contain the blueprint for health, we should do our best to preserve their energy; in particular, during severe illness we should avoid activities that drain them; we should concentrate on the aspects of Mercury that we tend to ignore most — i.e. rest and quiet; we should do things slowly, avoid that most Mercurial communication of all, sex, and avoid too much standing, lifting and work.

Syndromes of the Kidneys

1. Kidney yin deficiency;
2. Kidney yang deficiency;
3. Kidney jing deficiency;
4. Kidney qi not firm;
5. Kidney fails to grab the qi.

These are the basic syndromes; but the Kidneys also form important relationships with the four other zang, Liver, Heart, Spleen and Lungs, and these are discussed under those headings.

1. Kidney yin deficiency

If Kidney yin, which forms the basic blueprint of the body's yin, is deficient, then it is deficient in relation to Kidney yang. So Kidney yin deficiency has signs of yang, called 'empty' or 'false' yang.

Symptoms

(Note that very seldom will all be present simultaneously!)

(a) Vertigo and dizziness
     Noises in the head or ear (slow onset).
     Blurred vision
     Deafness
     Poor memory.
        These arise when Kidney fails to fill the 'Sea of Marrow'.
(b) Feverish or burning sensations in palms, soles, chest and ears
     Malar flush, worse after over-exertion
     Dry throat or mouth
     Thirst
     Sweating at night, not due to heat of room
     Constipation and dark urine
     Red tongue.
        Deficient yin fails to balance yang, leading to exhaustion of fluids. Feelings of heat and dryness are often worse in the afternoons.

(c) Nocturnal emissions; spermatorrhoea; because Kidney fails to store jing.

(d) General Kidney dysfunctions include:
Fear
Sore back, weak knees, deficient teeth or gums
Ringing in ears; deafness.

(e) General yin problems include:
Tendency towards restlessness, tension and unease
Emaciation or thinness
Desire for cool surroundings; a feeling of inner heat
High blood pressure
Sleeplessness.

The usual causes of Kidney yin deficiency are overwork over a long period; long illness which has severely drained the vitality; overindulgence in sex; acute febrile disease; prolonged haemorrhage; drugs, particularly those that boost yang. Overwork can be both lifting and standing; or too much brain work (which taxes the 'Sea of Marrow').

If false yang continues for too long, there may be increasing signs of heat as follows:

Great restlessness and unease
Mild fever
Continual waking from sleep, or insomnia
Priapism, nymphomania
Hot flushes, as at menopause
Dark, burning urine, smelling more strongly
Fast pulse.

The increased sexual desire reflects Kidney yang not being balanced by Kidney yin. The other symptoms derive from Empty Heat.

Kidney yin problems are often associated with such Western diseases as, for example, nervous excitement, hypermania, essential hypertension, as well as long standing ear and back problems. Not infrequently, a dry hot throat and mild fever is treated with antibiotics, which not only fail to eradicate a non-existent virus but which may further weaken Kidney yin. Equally, thirst can lead to a diagnosis of diabetes, or hypertension can lead to a prescription for tranquillizers. Western prescription may or may not mask the symptoms, but it is unlikely to cure them unless it deals with the root cause.

2. Kidney yang deficiency

Kidney yang carries the seed of all Fire in the body, so, if deficient, there is cold and fear of cold.

Symptoms

(a) Lumbar area feels cold, and aches.
   Legs are weak, especially knees, and may feel cold.
   (These areas are governed by the Kidneys).
(b) General aversion to cold. Limbs may be cold. Spine may feel cold.
   Facial pallor. Pulse deep, may be slow.
   (Here Kidney yang fails to warm).
(c) In man: impotence; premature ejaculation; seminal emission; sexual problems that can have a mental correlation.
   In woman: frigidity; sterility; no desire.
   (Kidney yang fails to warm Kidney jing.)
(d) Lassitude, apathy, a subdued behaviour
   Vertigo and confusion
   Pale tongue and weak pulse
   (Kidney yang fails to nourish Blood and muscles.)
(e) Loose stools: diarrhoea in early morning
   Urine clear and copious (usually)
   Cannot control urination: dribble
   Tongue swollen and may have teethmarks.
   (Kidney yang fails to 'move' or transform the fluids.)

Sometimes urine is clear but almost absent. When this occurs, there is also often oedema, which begins in the legs and ankles; here Kidney yang is particularly weak. But it might not appear in thin people until they are relatively old.

(f) General Kidney dysfunctions such as:
   Deafness, ringing in the ears
   Sore back, weak knees
   Fear. Fear with Kidney yang deficiency is less marked than with Kidney yin deficiency.

The usual causes are excess sex, prolonged illness and old age. But anything that weakens Spleen yang, which is supplied by Kidney yang, will eventually weaken Kidney yang. This would include poor food.

   The idea that problems can be caused by excess sex may seem

ridiculous to Westerners, but it is taken very seriously by traditional Chinese medicine. Excess sex relates not just to the constitution — some can perform prodigies of endurance and remain apparently healthy! — but to the state of health at the time and even to the time of year. So it is thought unwise to indulge too freely when tired or ill, or in winter time. It is better to enjoy sex in spring, and when feeling refreshed, say in the morning — at least from the man's point of view. (However, if he is of poor constitution but not too tired, the evening may be better; he has time to recuperate his energy overnight.) Not all women, however, are happy to wait until the morning. This seems to be something that Chinese medicine has not quite worked out yet, you may be relieved to hear! But the general caution regarding sex remains.

Because Kidney yang is the source of yang in the body, and because yang is moving and dispersing in nature, anything that weakens yang is to be avoided when undergoing treatment. This includes not only sex, but cold food and drink. Patients are advised to rest and keep warm. Even in summer they should avoid iced drinks and food, which may weaken Spleen yang, leading to retention of Damp, which, like a fog, retards movement of qi and yang, further weakening Kidney yang.

Deficient Kidney yang is diagnosed as many different diseases, including hypothyroidism, depression, neurasthenia, chronic urinary and kidney problems, deafness, lumbago and its frequently associated problems of sciatica.

3. Kidney jing deficiency
As this is a condition of emptiness of jing, the main problems concern reproduction and growth. Unless complicated with yin or yang syndromes, there are no signs of Hot or Cold syndromes.

(a) *Developmental*
    E.g. poor development of bones in children: poor tooth growth
    'Disease' due to physical/mental retardation
    Late puberty and menarche
    Weak Knees.
(b) *Sexual*
    Weak sexual powers.
(c) *Failure of Jing to feed the 'Sea of Marrow'*
    Poor memory (more important in adults)
    Dizziness
    Mental weakness or uncertainty
    Forcelessness and weak perseverance.

(d) *General*
Ear problems: deafness or tinnitus
Hair: falls or greys early
Circulation: poor
Weakness of other 'ancestral fu' (q.v.).
(e) *Kidney Yin problems*
E.g. Painful, sore back
Poor hearing
Teeth loose.

Causes: poor inherited constitution; chronic illness; shock; trauma in adults; old age.
    In adults there is less hope of rapid marked improvements on being correctly treated.

4. Kidneys fail to grasp qi
When we exhale, the lungs send qi down towards the Kidneys, which are said to receive and grasp or grab it. If the Kidney fails, we cannot easily inhale, since what is inhaled goes to them. This is particularly relevant in asthma, where a patient cannot inspire. To reach this stage, we must have drained our body of energy over a long period, during which we have continually demanded more output than is supplied by our food and air intake. The balance has come from our Kidney, energy which, as already explained, can be replenished only very slowly. Consequently there are many symptoms of deficiency.

Symptoms
Shortness of breath aggravated by exertion
Asthma — inhalation difficult. Breathing is fast but weak
Coughing
Sweating, coldness of limbs; thinness
Facial swelling — because Lungs cannot send qi downwards
Urination during asthmatic attack.
    It is noticeable that as we live in an ever faster-moving world, requiring more output and less regular eating and resting, we demand more of our Kidney energy. Hence this condition is increasingly common.

5. Kidney qi not firm
The area involved is the lower chou. If the Kidney is not firm, things escape through poorly latched portals; so besides general signs of

weak Kidney, there are urogenitary deficiency symptoms.

Symptoms
(a) *Urogenitary*
    Urinating with a weak force
    Dribbling urine between urinating; incontinence
    Urination while asleep
    Nocturnal emissions: spermatorrhoea
    Weak sexual performance: premature ejaculation
    Chronic vaginal discharges
    Prolapsed uterus.
(b) *General Kidney weakness*
    Sore back, tinnitus, deafness, loose teeth.

The causes of this are usually too much sex, especially early in life. Any strain on the lower chou can produce the same result; e.g. too many childbirths close together, or abortions. Old age is a contributory factor. The same situation can occur in young children as far as nocturnal enuresis is concerned. Here the Kidney energy has not yet 'firmed up'.

Path of Water Phase Channels
The Bladder channel starts at the inner corner of the eye. It ascends the forehead to the vertex, from where a branch runs to the temple. From the vertex it enters the brain, emerging at the back of the neck, from which two parallel lines run down either side of the spine, to the sacrum, one sending from the lumbar region a branch to the kidney and bladder organs, down through the gluteal muscles to the popliteal fossa. Here it meets the other branch which has proceeded over sacrum and posterior thigh. Together they descend the leg, circling posterior to the external malleolus to run along the outside edge of the foot to the small toe, linking with the Kidney meridian.

The Kidney meridian starts under the small toe, runs obliquely across the sole to the lower aspect of the tuberosity of the navicular bone, up behind the internal malleolus and into the heel. It then ascends along the medial side of the leg, the popliteal fossa and thigh to the vertebral column, from which it enters the kidney and bladder organs.

From the kidney it re-emerges, ascends through the liver and diaphragm, enters the lung, along the throat and ends at the root of the tongue.

From the lung a branch joins the heart, flows into the chest and links with the Pericardium channel.

Water phase imbalances often arise along these channels, e.g. on sole of foot, at the knee, in the spine and the bladder. Certain kinds of asthma and some throat and tongue problems also occur because they are on these channels. Equally, there are certain heavy, crushing headaches at the back of the head on the Bladder channel, which have a Water phase origin.

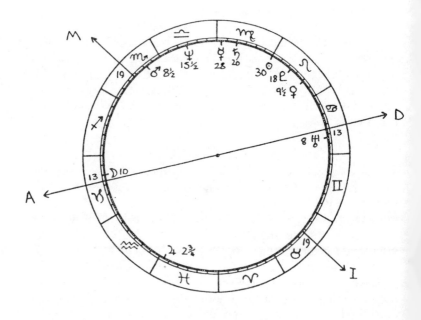

Chart 5. Male, 30.

Case 5: Male, 30; presenting complaint impotence
This chart is placed here to emphasize the importance of ♃ in problems of impotence; but it shows an almost unaspected ☿, which suggests weakness in Water.

'Weakness in Water' because of an unaspected ☿! This, surely, is hardly justified. But in terms of astrology, an unaspected planet is one that is not integrated, though its effect may be anything but weak. It may indeed be the most obvious thing about the person — in this case extreme nervousness (☿) and mental introspection; in the case of unaspected ♅ it might have been extreme independence, and so on. As such, its energy may be over-used at times, particularly if the planet ruling the phase that follows it is too strong, as here in the case of ♃. But we should never forget that to call something weak is only one way of looking at it; it is commonly said that the weakest link in the chain breaks first. An alternative view is that we show symptoms in our strongest energy phase, because that is the one that we rely on most, and which the other body energies look to for defence. Be that as it may, this chart is one of Wood overgrowth (♃), undernourished by the Water phase (☿).

Tall and nervous, desperately needing reassurance and mothering, we might say that he had outgrown his strength. His mother was a potent influence (☽ ☌ A); when she got ill, so did he, emotionally if not physically. He needed a job that cast him in the role of support (☽ 12, and most planets on the right side of the chart), yet he was ambitious (♄ A), although terrified of making a fool of himself, (☉ ☍ ♃, ☽ □ ♆). He was not especially good at making friends (♀ □ ♂), being so shy, and of course he chose as wife someone stronger than himself (☽ ☍ ♅ △ ♂) of whom he was frightened. But he was no fool, and in an unemotional atmosphere could be very capable, with an active imagination and good ability for progress. (Grand △ in Water signs, ♂, ♃, ♅). So his skills (☿) were not in doubt. His problem was not one of self-assertion: he could say what he wanted if necessary, and ♂ is well-placed and aspected. But if there was any doubt as to his belonging, his active mind (☿) produced paralysis. He never said as much, but the position of ♃ x suggests great imagination that perhaps over excited him, producing tension, and he had certainly masturbated too much in his past — i.e. abused his Kidney yin. The position of ☽ ♄ shows a strong need for a steady, reliable, orthodox lifestyle, with a nice home and good food, and he was unhappy in too challenging an environment. Yet ☽ ☍ ♅ points to a challenging parental influence, and astrologers will note the paucity of aspects to both ☿ and ♄, the latter also strongly indicative of parents, especially the father. He was terrified of his father, who had achieved great honour, but who was not an easy parent; yet he undoubtedly inherited persistence from him. But in a sexual role, his body refused to co-operate. The Moon's position in ♄, and the power of ♄, make it not surprising that he married fairly early. But when it came to initiating a new life, his ☿, ♃, ☽ and ♄ conspired against him. Specifically he was diagnosed as having depressed Liver qi, with some Kidney and Liver yin weakness leading to occasional signs of Liver yang: the effect was that Liver (Wood) overacted on Earth, and he had digestive problems, constipation, and inability to swallow food when eating with business colleagues. These digestive problems are not surprising with such a prominent ☽♑ ☍ ♅, but this is hardly enough to explain the impotence. For this we have to consider the ☿, ♄ and ♃. (☿) Water's deficiency leads to (♃) Wood's apparent excess (i.e. Liver yang). But ♄ (Earth) is not integrated enough to give the ability for calmness and easy reflection.

How to advise this man? Firstly he needed reassurance, and comfort that was not too directive or challenging. He needed to be able to talk without the feeling that he was being judged. He also probably needed a wife who was infinitely nurturing and mothering, but few women have the patience of a saint, and his wife was becoming restive after not a few years of marriage. He probably also needed more independence and trust in his good qualities at work. When first he came for treatment he was unhappy in his job, but eventually there was a change for the better. Meantime, whether because of treatment, or the gentle hand of a determined Nature, his Liver qi was flowing more smoothly, he was less nervous, his digestive problems were much better and he had a pregnant wife.

The Four Phases: Reconsideration

Wood, Fire, Metal, Water is a natural process of growth, maturity, decay and rest, which each of us enjoys daily and yearly. But each phase has many aspects. For example, the Wood phase governs the ability of the body to replenish its reserves during rest, for growth is useless without reserves. Wood may be expansion and Metal decay; but with the expired breath we expel rubbish our body no longer needs, and we send qi to all the other organs. Wood cannot grow without that qi; the quiet rest of the Water phase would be terminal without it! And a fire without air goes out. So each phase assists every other phase to some extent.

Water is the blueprint phase, when we rest and adjust our bodies to the day's stress. Failure here comes from chronic disease and over-exertion without adequate rest, and leads to a general weakness according to Kidney yin or yang. If yang is weak we are cold: if yin is weak we are hot. So Kidney yang contains the germ of all heat in the body, and Kidney yin nourishes but controls overgrowth, by providing an anchor for it. If Kidney yin is weak, we suffer from an

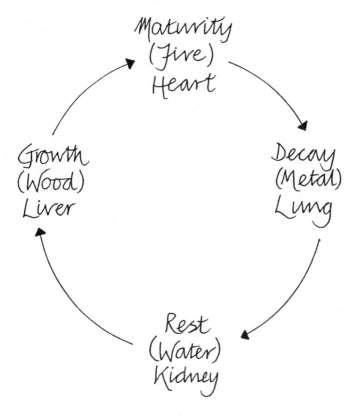

Diagram 5.

overabundance of yang in the growth of Wood and the abundance of Fire. In the above diagram, the Water phase that supplies Wood and Fire is predominantly yin.

Yin is therefore nourishment, decay and rest (Metal, Water); yang is growth, movement and warmth (Wood, Fire). When yang is blocked, we get frustration, tension, pain, loss of self-confidence and loss of joy. If yin is blocked, we lose the ability to rest, to recoup our energy and to reflect and meditate. Toxins build up and we poison ourselves. There is often a build-up of mucus and cattarh, which is assumed to be a chronic 'cold'.

Case 6: Female, 29
We can begin to consider a rather more complicated chart. Notice the important planets are all fairly powerful:

♅   ♂A♋
☉   Highest placed in sky
☿   No aspects save ▢.☍
♇   Only planet placed in 1st quadrant.

If we accept that ♇ is co-ruler with ☿ of Water phase, then there are two important pointers to a Fire-Water and to a yin-yang imbalance; one is unaspected ☿; the other the strong, although difficult, position of ♇ (which is opposite the area of the chart it rules in Western astrology) ▢☉▢.♂: two moving, dispersing and warming planets in aspect with the slowest-moving and deepest-working planet of all. This might suggest a hereditary problem to do with growth and movement. This perhaps is backed up by the position of ♅♂A giving an independent and perhaps determinedly 'different' personality.

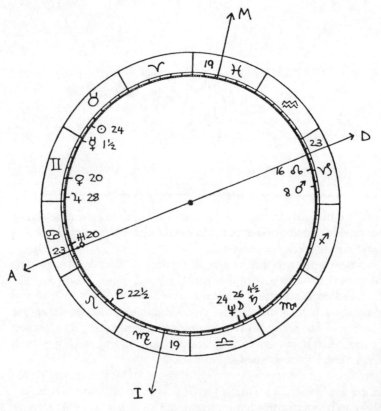

Chart 6. Female, 29.

The other pointer towards a weakness at the base of the energy is the ☽ ♆ conjunction at the base of the chart, square Ascendant.

Going no further than this, we might deduce some long-term strain on the yin phases, in particular Water, since ☿ and ♇ are both uncomfortable. Given that ☿ ♊ will always find a way out, this lady is unlikely to run out of ideas or things to do. She will have a quick, perceptive mind and a good versatility. From this we see that as ☿ rules the Water phase, and Kidneys give skill and techniques, so also does ☿ associate with Geminian adaptability and manual dexterity.

We can look on her good brain and ability for skilful manual technique as either being derived from Kidney (which rules skill and technique) or from ☿ ruling Gemini. In either case, ☿ is involved. (Of course there are other reasons too, such as ♅ ☌ A; but I hope to show later how ♅ derives its energy from ☿ in Chinese medicine in the same way as, in Western astrology, ♅ is said to be a higher plane of ☿.)

The position of ♂ lends it prominence by being the only planet in the area between ☉ and ♄. From here it may be said to balance all the other planets; but it does so from a yin area of the chart, because the planet is receding from the top of the chart, and has passed the Descendant. We might therefore expect it to work somewhat erratically, able neither to project Fire nor to balance Water. From its position we might also guess lower middle or lower chou problems of over-heating: ♂ in a yin area of the chart ⚼ ♇, a very yin planet, and ☉ a very yang planet.

In terms of character, we expect someone of considerable inner strength and fortitude who works hard and willingly in her chosen areas but who is let down by feelings of fear and a lack of self-assurance; she doesn't feel good enough. She may also seek to boost the energy of her lower chou with drugs that assist (initially, they later destroy) lower chou energy, or sex, which give feelings of power and strength. Her desire for exploration of new experiences should be strong (♅ ☌ A; ☿ ♊, etc.).

So, drawing the threads together, we expect a weakness in the Water phase, and also a weakness of yang (because ♂ is somewhat weak, and the ☉ weakened by difficult aspects to ♆ and ☽). In addition, we perhaps expect signs of heat in the lower chou, the area of greatest weakness. We also expect the problems that arise from too exploratory a spirit which makes errors of judgement (♅ ☌ A), and which lacks a sense of belonging (☽ ♆ □ A) to a secure way of life. There will be a feeling of fear, carefully guarded.

She came for treatment at 29, with P☉ = 22° ♓; P☽ =

23° ♏(Δ☽); P☿ = 16°♋ P♀ = 26°♋; P♂ = 5½° ♑ ᴿ; P♃ = 4½°♋; P♄ = 3° ♏; T♇ = 2° ♏; T♆ 0° ♑; T♅ = 12° ♐; T♄ = 15° ♏; T♃ = 0° ♑; T♂ = 5° ♏; i.e. T♂ + ♇ ♂ ♇ ♄. She had kidney area pains on her back which had begun at 27, after a period when from the age of 23 she had had two abortions and one miscarriage. She was in low health, tired, and had many boils on her skin. At 27 she contracted an undiagnosed urinary infection which was not cystitis. This gave her excruciating pain on both sides of her abdomen. Antibiotics helped but the problem kept recurring. At 29, she felt the pain in her back if she drank much alcohol, and if she got cold or tired. It felt better for warmth and yoga. She was occasionally dizzy, and her circulation was poor, with hands and feet getting cold very easily. Her chest was tightened up by cold air, and she could not catch her breath or breathe in easily. (As a child she had had bad wheezing that was worse in cold weather and after certain foods and after exertion. She caught jaundice at 7.) Her heart area gave a fluttery feeling and she got hot if fearful. Her periods from the age of 15 became painful and she was put on the Pill, which made no difference. The pain was always on the first day of her period. At 19 she became pregnant and subsequently gave birth to a boy, after which she had feelings as if her uterus was prolapsing. After abortions at 23 and 25, and a miscarriage at 27, she had a second child at 28. She was made very tired by both babies. At night when asleep she gets very hot and sweats profusely, though she is not aware of this. As a child she was very frightened of her parents, who argued a lot. The fear continues even now when they argue, and affects her heart area.

There are signs here of Kidney deficiency. For example:

1. Kidney area pains worse for alcohol, cold and tiredness
   Kidney area pains better for heat, massage and yoga
   (Both of these Kidney yang)
2. Dizziness (Kidney yin)
   Chest: dyspnoea (Kidney cannot grab qi)
   Night flushes and sweats (Kidney yin)
   Heart area discomfort if nervous, and gets hot (Kidney and Heart yin)
   Poor circulation (Kidney yang)

On her father's side was a family history of 'weak' chests and deep red complexions, suggesting a Heart-Lung inherited deficiency. On the mother's side, there was a family history of cancer.

There is insufficient space to give a fuller discussion of the midpoints of this chart, but P = A/M and at the point when she contracted the original infection at 27, TP = 24°♎, TΨ = 24° ♐, T♅Ϊ = 0° ♐, T♄ = 17°♎, T♃ = 2° ♏, T♂ = 26°♎. If we take ☽ to represent the 'fabric' of the body and its natural processes, we see considerable strain due to these transiting planets, and T♅Ϊ ☍ ☿ᵣ, giving sudden changes and challenges to her ingenuity and life skills. (She was abroad at the time.) The preceding period from 23 to 27 began with P☽ ♂I.C., and T♄ ♂ P ᵣ. During this period she underwent two abortions and one miscarriage (as well as an accident when she fell from a bicycle). These would have further strained her jing.

If we look again at her chart, we see that it is in fact the chart of a highly Scorpionic person, which is how she seemed: strong and self-sufficient. But that strength was not won lightly! One wonders how she will go on, now that she has substantially overcome the temptations of the lower side of Scorpio and Pluto. Perhaps ♅Ϊ will lead her into some interesting new area where her experience can help others.

6.

SATURN ♄

Western astrology's major malefic has a lot to answer for. He forces us to face the essential necessities of life, the obligations to our parents, clan and race we acquire just by being born, and the responsibilities we have to accept if we wish to continue in existence. These responsibilities are sometimes taken over by the State, which succours the needy, provides a pension in old age, and, in some countries, a health insurance service for when our bodies let us down. No wonder we get a bit fed up with Saturn; what he requires from us is hard work and attention. He represents our body and its needs, though we are apt to confuse him with our creditors, who supplied our requirements.

But he represents more than our sustenance. Our bodies are where we live, and they carry a link in a chain that stretches back to the amoeba. All those ancient forefathers now lie dead, their bodies absorbed back into the earth, the atoms that made them now either minerals or new forms of food and life. We think of Saturn as being the reaper of lives; but he is the vehicle of life too. Without that physical vehicle, we die. He gives us shape and form; he gives us a family, parents and descendants, all links in the chain of being. And he demands that we keep that chain in being. So we must eat, guard our health and procreate. To do so we must plan and decide (♃), but avoid excess; learn to assert ourselves (♂) but never demand absolute control, save self-control. We must refine our experience, improve and purify ourselves (♀), not clinging to the apparent security of what we no longer require; and we must be ready to learn, adapt and rest (☿), letting sleep remove in oblivion our fears, anxieties and fatigue.

Whatever aspect of work leads to the continuation of the race and its safety comes under ♄. Our income in so far as it goes towards keeping us alive and well comes under ♄ and so does the food we eat and the exercise we take. Saturn is not very demanding really; he actually prefers the bare necessities: simple, uncontaminated food eaten regularly; a clean environment; adequate clothing, physical exertion and pure air; somewhere to live, neither too hot nor too cold; a supporting community or family. He is not interested in the big things of life, but if mankind is to continue he demands that we defend our needs and the structure of our integrity. He asks us to live safely and securely, and to achieve a society where his needs can continue to be met. Hence we must meet the approval of our peers by toeing the line, doing our bit, persisting.

And when we have achieved what ♄ demands, we find that we have grown old, and he no longer needs us alive in the flesh. So the flesh ceases to be a suitable place to live; it returns to the dust from whence it came.

Saturn always has the long term in mind. He is only interested in maintaining a vehicle for life. So as we store things up for the future we obey his call. Our pension, our savings and our store cupboard are eloquent witness to the importance we give to him; and if we forget him for too long, either he reminds us of our obligations, ruthlessly, or we die. Because of those long-term goals, we save, we strengthen ourselves and we acquire power over the future, but this is not really Saturn's responsibility. He does not ask us to become powerful at our friend's expense; if we do so it may be out of fear or ambition. He simply demands that we keep things going: that we are responsible. He is the voice of duty, calling us to maintain the plan.

Where we rebel, he will remind us, and modern psychological insight shows how often he is that part of ourselves that we least like, our shadow figure, reminding us of that aspect of our personality that needs attention. We may even see him as an enemy, personified usually by an associate we dislike, reminding us both outwardly and inwardly of the community we live in and all the individuals who make it up; like them or not, they are our companions and without them we should be poorer.

Astrologers look on the position and aspects of ♄ in a chart as showing the area of life in which there is likely to be some form of restriction, or discipline, and in which effort may have to be made. It configures the family, or racial, demand for survival in the flesh, and can be looked upon as the karmic inheritance from our predecessors, showing how we have to continue the burden and the enigma of life.

In Western astrology, Saturn is said to rule the bones, skin and teeth, the process of ossification, the problems of ageing, hardened arteries and all problems of blockage, to name but a few of its associations. In traditional Chinese medicine the emphasis is on the Blood and everything it nourishes, and on the process of transportation of material about the body. We have to see it as all the forms in which life manifests, and in particular in the supply of nutrition to all those different forms, whether they be bone, brain or inner organ. Although each form may 'belong' to one of the other orbs of energy (i.e. Heart, Liver, Kidney, Lung) the central flow of being towards it comes from Saturn. No wonder Saturn is blamed for degeneration and loss of vital organs. But this occurs either when we grow old, or when we fail to observe Saturn's requirements, by abusing ourselves. In the ordinary way Saturn gives life, not death.

Western medicine is only beginning to understand the function of the spleen organ. *Spleen* has always been of central importance in Chinese medicine, together with its associated organ, the *Stomach*. Spleen is ruled by Saturn.

Functions of Spleen

1. Spleen neutralizes, calms and integrates the polar energies of the other four zang

This shows how Spleen acts as an anchor for the other energies, which it irrigates and moistens. As the base in which the others operate, Spleen is central, overlooking and regulating the movement of all solids and liquids, as well as qi. The earth in which they operate gives birth to all. So if the central neutralizing, calming function is healthy, the other organs will find small reason for disease; they will be adequately nourished and able to communicate with one another. Understanding this is central to an understanding of Spleen function.

2. Spleen governs transformation and transportation

(a) *Transformation*
Food enters Stomach in which, together with Small Intestine, the energy of food is assimilated. This energy splits into two parts. One part goes to Lungs, where it mixes with qi from air, forming the energy that flows in the meridians and the energy that passes through all the organs, 'leading the blood' we might say. The other part is divided in Spleen, a 'pure' part going to energize each of the organs individually (i.e. Heart, Spleen itself, Lungs, Kidney and Liver), another part condensing to form fluids that

moisten Lung and Kidneys, another part going to moisten the skin, and a last part travelling to form a coating on the tongue ('moss').

Blood is also formed in Stomach and is sent initially to Liver for storage.

From the above we see how important is Stomach: it is paired with Spleen and controlled by Spleen, but whereas Stomach qi moves down (otherwise we should be nauseous or sick, and suffer from regurgitation and mucus) Spleen qi holds internal organs up or in place (failing which we suffer from prolapse and haemorrhoids, for example) as part of its job of providing the ground for life to function. When Spleen fails to transform we get a full, distended abdomen, with loose stools, belching, nausea and undigested food in the faeces, not to mention a lost appetite. These are basically symptoms of weak Spleen qi (see below).

(b) *Transportation*

Spleen directs energy and blood around and throughout the body. Where it fails, the organs and limbs are unable to obtain adequate nutrition, so feel heavy, tired, and eventually cold. The meridian cannot function without this energy, and muscles, skin and teeth cannot grow or be repaired.

Part of this job of transportation concerns movement of fluids around the body. In failure we get mucus in the intestines, oedema and even cellulitis. The problem of damp and mucus will arise later in the discussion, as they are very important. Here it should just be noted that mucus that arises because of a weak Spleen can affect mental as well as physical levels — giving mental woolliness, depression, confusion and insomnia.

A healthy Spleen gives a good appetite, an untroubled and reliable digestive process, adequate nourishment and normal transmission of fluids.

3. Spleen contains Blood

Once the Blood has been manufactured, Spleen maintains its circulation to all parts and prevents it escaping from the blood vessels: i.e. containment. This function is very close to the function of Heart in controlling Blood. But whereas Heart gives movement to Blood, Spleen provides the Blood and keeps it in order. Whereas Heart keeps order throughout the body through Blood, as befits Heart's function as Sovereign Prince, Spleen, on the other hand, is more like a Minister of Domestic Affairs: he is closer to the common people. But whereas the people look to him to maintain law and order, it is to their Prince, the Heart, that they bear allegiance. He it is who inspires them, and gives a direction to the organism's outer efforts; but it is Spleen who gets things done at home.

4. Spleen dominates flesh and muscles
The flesh and muscles receive nourishment from Spleen to enable them to grow strong and work. It is the substance and quality of the flesh that is meant, not its motor movement. So where Spleen fails we get emaciation and weariness. (Movement of muscles due to contraction comes under Liver.)

5. Spleen opens into the mouth
The mouth is the sense organ governed by Spleen: its health is shown by the state of the mouth and lips, and by the ability to receive and process food.

6. Spleen rules mental faculties of Concentration, Memory and Cogitation
These are the characteristics of calm reflection; the ability to think, to distinguish, essential in creative imagining. 'Read, mark, learn and inwardly digest' as the old saying has it, points out the relationship between mental and physical absorption. To do either properly we need to be grounded comfortably with ourselves. Where we lose that calm centre, we become obsessed, we take flights of fancy, we lose touch with reality, we can't think clearly. Over-use of the mind can bring us to this state, as when we work too hard for an exam, or grapple too long with a problem: our brain grows tired and confused and we need rest, sleep, a change. Failing this, our minds get stuck, as if in a fog. This is the mental equivalent of phlegm, which is produced when a weak Spleen fails to transform, or 'resolve' a fluid situation.

7. Spleen governs sympathy and affections
By affections is meant the feeling states of sympathy, consideration for others, and empathy. These are the deeper human values of civilization. The Fire phase may give the excitement of LOVE, but Earth phase gives a community and a family in which love can flourish. And when love becomes fondness, Earth gives a common interest and bond.

The stomach and spleen organs are situated in the middle chou (under the diaphragm and above the umbilicus) and this is the area governed by Spleen. The liver, also situated here, has a considerable influence on the middle chou, on Spleen and on the feeling states governed by Spleen. Together, Liver and Spleen control sympathy and antipathy, like and dislike, desire and revulsion. Astrologers will realize how important ♃ is in opening us to new experience, and ♄ is in channelling our energies to the essentials. We are given assertion and self-discipline by ♂, while ♀ gives consideration and value. But ♀ can also cut us off from our friends, and Metal phase, ruled by ♀, is frequently imbalanced when we cling to old relationships, thereby stopping development of new ones. So we cannot say that only Liver (Wood, ♃) and Spleen (Earth, ♄) are responsible for these feelings. If these middle chou energies are at peace and in balance, then self-assertion (♂) and self-evaluation (♀), joy and pleasure will arise naturally. If this centre is obsessed, or curdled round a clotted centre, how can we live in harmony with others?

In this connection should be mentioned the effects of shock; shock affects Heart first, but is said to lodge in Spleen. Shock can arise from many kinds of trauma, physical and emotional. If its effects have penetrated very deeply, then the central harmonizing spleen cannot function and one or more of the other phases may imbalance. In astrological terms we need to ensure that Saturn gives steadiness to the nature and, if it is weak, it may be helpful to cultivate steady pursuits to do with survival on an earthly level, such as gardening, body massage, cooking and clerical or manual jobs that anchor us to reality. (We might expect to see shock of this kind more in people of an emotional disposition, probably more feminine type than masculine type, therefore more commonly in women. Values are changing in some societies, where women are assertively enjoying more 'masculine' type behaviour than men. In these cases, and in the cases of masculine type people, commonly men, we might argue that the Moon's strength in a chart is most important for balance. In other words, as individuals develop femininity, they need the groundedness of duty, forbearance and discipline in Earth pursuits ruled by Saturn; as they go for a more masculine type behaviour, they put more of a strain on maternal and instinctual parts of their personality, sometimes confusing life instinct (☽) with selfish impulse (♂). This is rather to fly a kite: what is certain is that shock lodges in the Spleen!)

8. Other associations

(a) *Dryness; coolness.*
    Whereas a warm damp environment is best for Stomach energy,

Spleen prefers dryness and coolness so that impure qi can condense. The warm damp is necessary for the stomach to 'rotten and ripen', i.e. digest, its contents. But the qi that emerges from this process needs coagulating and this needs a cooler atmosphere. Too much damp or mucus-forming food will inhibit Spleen function. Such foods include dairy products, often at fault where there is a lot of mucus.

(b) *Uterus and breasts*

Spleen plays a major part in the functioning of these organs. The uterus in particular is the 'ground' in which new life develops. Nourishment here must be finely calculated: it must be the best. An irregular diet in the mother, with drugs and poor living habits, will strain Spleen's ability to feed the foetus what it needs. The uterus is what makes the woman — her most precious part, where she creates life; the centre of her being. It grounds her in her physical function and there is, in traditional Chinese medicine, a direct relationship, via a special channel, between uterus and heart. Many cases of dysmenorrhoea and even menorrhagia are due to dysfunction in Liver, Heart and Spleen energies, yet it is the uterus which is surgically removed, one of the most yin of all organs. Is it not surprising that hysterectomies so often produce women with deficiency in Heart or Liver yin syndromes? It is as if their ♄ had been torn out, and they cannot settle with themselves: they become restless and over-emotional. Worse still, their problems, which were once physical, become more prominent on a mental level, with anxiety and pain for which Western medicine can discover no physical basis. They are diagnosed 'psychosomatic' and given tranquillizers; not infrequently the same drug that they received before the operation. (This is not to suggest that hysterectomies are always a bad thing, but that they are prescribed too frequently, and for problems that traditional Chinese medicine at least can often treat.)

The role of ♄ in the charts of women who are infertile, or who for some reason are unable to bear children, is often indicative of a reluctance to be the ground in which life will grow, and correlates with a personality that chooses either a lifestyle that is incompatible with childbearing — it may be overworked or over-caring for others — or a spouse who is unwilling or unable to fertilize her. In this latter respect ♄ takes on a traditional role and represents the woman's father/husband with whom there may have been a difficult bond, or who may have had some form of hidden weakness. If the role of earning money to support the family is seen as that of the traditional male, then we may have a connection, represented by ♄ in a chart, between the father who doubts himself (say), whose seed produces a girl child who lacks a sure sense of self-identity, who then gives herself up in some self-sacrificial way, and whose Blood lacks the substance to produce children. Lacking yin, she may be prone to panic — which can abort a child if conceived. (That women with this configuration can and do conceive is not in doubt: we are discussing only a tendency. Besides, there are other reasons for infertility.)

The breasts are governed by Spleen, but Liver energy is also important for smooth flow of qi through them, and when a woman's breasts are swollen and painful before her period, the usual culprit is Liver overacting on Spleen (Wood overacts on Earth). This overacting is derived usually from either deficient Liver yin or stuck Liver.

Sound
People with Spleen imbalance sometimes speak in a rather singsong voice, rather as one might use to a child.

Odour
'Fragrant'; a very sweet and rather sickly smell, sometimes also noticeable in people who have eaten too well the night before, or who drink too much gin, whisky or vodka, or in pre-menstrual women. (In each of these examples, Spleen energy is strained, and we should expect to find other signs of Spleen imbalance. For example, those who drink too much alcohol may also suffer from skin ulcers, where pus (mucus) builds up in the flesh because Spleen qi is weakened. But in such a case we should probably also find signs of internal Heat.)

Taste
'Sweet'; ideally this sweetness is the taste of well-chewed grain and not that of sugar. If we remember that Spleen governs the transformation of food into qi then we realize why sugar and other sweet foods are often so attractive to one whose Spleen is weak. Sugar is like qi: it gives a quick boost, but it is short-lived and encourages a lazy Spleen, so blood sugar levels go up and down fast and we want more sugar. Sugar rots the teeth, which are governed in general by Spleen (since they lie in the mouth, though there is a still closer

relationship between Kidney and teeth); so we see how raw sugar, or any sweet substance, opposes Spleen action on several levels. Sugar, by weakening Spleen qi, creates dampness (see below).

Functions of Stomach

Earth phase energy contains Spleen and Stomach. Because Stomach is so basic in the formation of qi and Blood, it is the only zangfu organ/official to be described in detail in this book. For convenience, and because their energies are so closely interconnected, the pair are often called Spleen/Stomach. This means that no clear distinction is made between them in practice. Another reason for including Stomach is that the path of the Stomach meridian lies entirely on the yin, anterior, surface of the body; no other yang meridian has this. One surmises that this is because Stomach's role is so important in producing nutritive (yin) energy, whereas the other yang organs (Colon, Small Intestine, Bladder, Gall Bladder) are less central to this.

1. Stomach rottens and ripens food
It receives, temporarily stores, and digests food. Acting as an energy reservoir, it sends energy to the other officials.

2. Stomach qi descends
When it fails, we have nausea, regurgitation, and a build-up of mucus in nose and throat, often noticeable after a big meal.

3. Stomach requires a warm damp environment
This means for adequate digestion the stomach lining should be warm and damp. Hence it may be unwise to swallow quantities of ice-cold liquid or food if there is any weakness in digestion. Likewise, food that heats and dries out the stomach can be injurious, such as spicy food that is too hot, or alcohol that is too potent or too much.

Syndromes of Spleen

Syndromes of Spleen may be divided into two categories: first, weak qi of Spleen; and secondly, invasion of Spleen by Cold Damp. The former has four types:

1. Weak Spleen qi
2. Sinking Spleen qi
3. Dysfunction in Blood containment
4. Spleen yang deficiency.

1. Weak Spleen qi

Weakness of Spleen means hypofunction of Spleen and its related tissues and organs.

Sallow complexion, often emaciation
Anorexia
Abdominal distension. Stuffiness in chest
Oedema — usually of legs and arms
Loose stools
General lassitude
Tongue is pale: moss white: pulse slippery or thready.

Usual causes

(a) 'Irregular' food intake, i.e. eating too little, too often, too much; eating unusual food; eating in a hurry, etc. Voracious eating is especially harmful, and often occurs on holiday (together with a Stomach syndrome), when illness is blamed on unaccustomed germs or viruses in the food.

(b) Excess mental strain, or excessive exertion. By excessive is meant extreme exertion or strain over a long period. But it cannot help to return to work too soon after eating, or to eat while working.

(c) *Protracted chronic disease damages Spleen qi*
Physiologically, weak Spleen qi — weakened transformation and transportation — mainly reflects on intestinal function, leading to disturbances in absorption and distribution and increased fluid in the intestines, anorexia, abdominal distension and loose stools. An old Chinese saying is that 'Spleen weakness produces damp; excess damp leads to loose stools.'

Note: oedema can be caused by dysfunction of Lung, Spleen and Kidney. Only the above symptoms point to weak Spleen qi.

2. Sinking Spleen qi

This is a further development of weak Spleen qi and is from protracted chronic disease causing general weakness.

Symptoms

Almost always there are symptoms of weak Spleen qi. Bearing down sensation in abdominal area, especially, around the umbilicus: shortness of breath; prolapse of e.g. rectum, uterus, stomach, intestine.

These conditions are called 'Sinking Spleen qi' because the

symptoms are in the lower part of the body, and because the Spleen fails to hold internal organs in place; hence they move downwards. If the sensation of bearing down improves on lying down, then there is usually prolapse. Prolapse is often better in good health and after rest, worse after exertion and in ill health. The causes are the same as for weak Spleen qi, but extend over a longer period.

3. Dysfunction in Blood containment
All kinds of haemorrhage, accompanied by symptoms of weak Spleen qi, e.g. purpura, bloody stool, and uterine bleeding.

(It should be noted that purpura (for example) is caused by other conditions than weak Spleen: 'Heat in the Blood (q.v.) and allergies are also factors.) In weak Spleen dysfunction in Blood containment, the bleeding occurs usually in lower parts of the body, as one would expect from a Spleen that is too weak to hold things up and in place. So haematemesis and nose bleeds are usually due to other factors impinging on and weakening Spleen function locally.

4. Spleen yang deficiency
This usually comes from extreme weakness of Spleen qi.

Symptoms
Signs of weak Spleen qi are chilliness and cold extremities.

Prolonged Spleen qi weakness leads to weakness of defensive qi, which is unable to warm the superficial layers of the body; hence the chilliness. Spleen yang qi also transports nourishment and warmth to the extremities; if it fails, they grow cold.

Invasion of Spleen by Cold Damp

Symptoms
    Stuffiness in chest and epigastrium
    Anorexia
    Heavy sensation in head
    General lassitude
    Borborygmous
    Abdominal pain and loose stool
    Tongue: moss white and sticky
    Pulse: thready or soft or slippery.

Whereas the other Spleen syndromes are due to deficiency, this is caused by invasion of 'cold Damp' which damages Spleen qi. It is therefore a problem of 'excess', at least initially. However, if untreated, or even mistreated, the excess may remain, further weakening Spleen qi, so that in practice one often sees symptoms of weak Spleen qi accompanied by symptoms of excess 'Cold Damp invasion'.

Some of these symptoms are similar to weak Spleen qi. We distinguish them by two main criteria: (1) different causative factors; (2) duration.

Included under causative factors is invasion from exterior to interior of 'cold damp', e.g. exposure to cold or damp conditions, such as being caught in the rain, living in a damp basement, sitting on wet grass.

The other causative factor is invasion of Cold Damp through the mouth due to improper food intake e.g. eating frozen or iced food, watermelon and fruit when the stomach is weakened or unready. The Chinese seldom eat raw food and one reason is that they fear invasion of Cold Damp. (The fact that in their preference for hot food they cook in too much oil, causing heat and eventually phlegm, which then weakens Spleen qi, shows that they can suffer from over-enthusiasm!) Ice cream in particular, being cold, damp and sweet, can have a devastating effect on Spleen energy. Like all cold or raw foods, it should be preceded by warm foods or drinks. This warms the stomach, enabling it to cope.

Those who have weak Spleens, or who have suffered a prolonged period of poor health, are usually advised to begin their meals with warm food, and to reduce intake of cold food. In summer, we tend to eat more cool food, but over-indulgence in iced food can quickly produce symptoms of cold damp in those who have a pre-disposition towards weak Spleen qi. Such people are discussed under the chapter on yin and yang; here we may simply say that older people are more susceptible.

As to the question of duration, symptoms of invasion by Cold Damp usually take place within a few days, whereas symptoms of Spleen qi deficiency develop gradually.

Invasion of Cold Damp from exterior to interior occurs through the skin. Damp is characterized by heaviness, so leads to obstruction of qi in the gastro-intestinal system, and heaviness of chest or epigastrium. If damp invades via the skin, some of it may remain at superficial level, in muscles and tissues, giving a heavy sensation of the whole body or a sensation in the head that feels like a heavy 'hat', or as if wrapped up in something. Where damp invades the superficial muscles and tissues (tendino-muscular system in traditional Chinese medicine) it can remain for a considerable time, causing local stiffness which is better for continued movement. The stiffness is sore and feels bruised; in acute symptoms there is restlessness, and the first movement (from a state of rest) is usually painful. It is often described as rheumatism in Western medicine. It is better for heat, rubbing and movement. Nowadays cyclists with low-slung handlebars on their cycles tend to get this condition in their backs after exposure to rain and damp.

Dampness is more fully discussed in Chapter 9, 'Origins of Disease'. It should be added that Damp Heat can also invade Spleen. It occurs usually when we eat contaminated food, and the symptoms are much the same as for Cold Damp, but there are signs of heat — such as a sweet, sticky taste in the mouth, mild fever, dry mouth and lips; moss on the tongue is yellow or greasy.

Syndromes of Stomach

The main syndromes are:

1. Heat in Stomach;
2. Cold in Stomach;
3. Stagnant qi in Stomach;
4. Congealed Blood in Stomach;
5. Stomach yin deficiency;
6. Mucus in Stomach.

1. Heat in Stomach
In increasing severity, there is:

(a) dryness, thirst for excessive quantities of cold fluids;
(b) great hunger, foul breath, nausea after eating, belching, epigastric burning pain, mental agitation;
(c) toothache, gums swollen, inflamed, bleeding, constipation, irritability, red face.

Pulse is fast and slippery, big or flooding. Tongue is red; moss is thick, dry and yellow. Usual causes are:

(a) too much hot, spicy, greasy food or alcohol;
(b) Liver Fire invading stomach;
(c) Heat in Stomach out of harmony with Cold in Spleen.

2. Cold in Stomach
Epigastric pain that is mildly cramping and persistent. Epigastric or abdominal swelling. Likes heat, massage and warm food. Worse cold. Has little energy. May have heartburn. Walking makes fluids swish around inside.

If Stomach qi rebels there will also be nausea, vomiting or hiccups. Vomiting, if it occurs, is of watery fluid, and makes the patient feel better. Tongue is pale; moss is white and sticky; pulse is slow or thready.

This condition is due to invasion of cold, eating or drinking cold things. Such cold directly or indirectly injures yang of Stomach, leading to weakness of Stomach in digesting food normally. Weak Stomach yang leads to weak Spleen yang because Spleen and Stomach are related.

3. Stagnant qi in Stomach
Stomach ache with abdominal distension, the pain sometimes extending to the side of the ribs. Flatulence. Some belching. Headaches. Sour taste in mouth. Tongue either normal or dark, tinged purple at sides. Pulse wiry. Symptoms are often caused by emotional factors, worry and tension; there is usually an irritable nature.

4. Congealed Blood in Stomach
Stabbing pain in epigastrium; may feel lumpy; worse for touch; complexion and stools are dark; patient looks and feels ill; vomit contains blood; pulse rough and wiry; tongue is dark with red spots; moss is thin and yellow. Usually due to longstanding strain on Spleen Stomach, e.g. worry, anxiety, or invasion of Earth by Wood with concomitant tension, over a long period. Also due to Heat, e.g. Liver Fire, possibly aggravated by intake of heating substances such as alcohol, greasy or fried foods and drugs. This condition sometimes develops out of stagnant Stomach qi.

5. Stomach yin deficient
Because Stomach yin consists of the fluids and mucus in the stomach, in deficiency there is dryness with difficulty swallowing, anorexia, difficulty digesting; vomit is dry; dry stools, usually constipated. There is often pain, often due to an ulcer. Mentally there is a kind of weak nervous emaciation. Tongue is dry, may peel; usually red or scarlet. Pulse thin and fast.

This condition occurs as the end result of an outside evil, with heat injuring the Stomach, and is associated with chronic conditions like a poor lifestyle and poor eating habits, for example eating too much or too late at night.

6. Mucus in Stomach hangs and collects
Dizziness, much phlegm and a heavy lethargic condition; symptoms

are close to Spleen qi deficiency. Usually there is either anorexia or ravenous hunger, and a rather depressed attitude to life. Tongue is pale; moss is greasy and dirty; and pulse is slippery. This condition often arises in overweight patients, because they are said to have 'excess dampness', a Chinese euphemism for 'fat'. The condition can arise when Spleen qi is weak, but can be due to too much rich food and insufficient exercise.

Path of Earth Phase Meridians

The Stomach channel starts beside the nose, ascends to the bridge of the nose, then down the face to the upper gums, the lips, across the jaw and up to the lateral forehead at the hairline. From the jaw it runs down the neck to the supraclavicular fossa; then on down through the diaphragm to stomach and spleen organs. On the surface it runs vertically down through the nipple, past the umbilicus to the lower abdomen just lateral to the pubic bone. The channel continues down the anterior aspect of the thigh, lateral to the patella to the leg, ankle and second and third toes, sending a branch to the large toe, where it becomes the Spleen channel.

The Spleen channel starts from the large toe, runs along the medial aspect of the foot at the junction of red and white skin, in front of the internal malleolus and up the medial leg, knee and thigh to the abdomen, where it enters the spleen and stomach. It ascends through the diaphragm beside the oesophagus to the root of the tongue and its lower surface. From the stomach it sends a branch into the heart.

From this we see, for example, that some pains connected with Spleen/Stomach problems occur on the anterior aspect of the leg; likewise many sinus pains in the head occur on the Stomach meridian.

7.

YIN AND YANG

Traditional Chinese Medicine and Macrobiotics

These are of fundamental importance in appreciating traditional Chinese medicine, and it is to the credit of Georges Ohsawa and his philosophy of Macrobiotics that they have almost passed into the common usage. Unfortunately, they are much misunderstood. Still more unfortunate is the fact that yin and yang as used in Macrobiotics are different in several vital ways from their use in Chinese medicine. They are similar in that in both systems they convey a polar quality of effects: neither can be comprehended without some reference to the other. It is ridiculous to speak of an article's size without comparing it with another. Consider the following:

'Dad, how big is a battleship?'
'What sort of battleship, Son?'
'A big one, Dad.'
'How big, Son?'

Each side of the equation of yin and yang connects with the other side, and not only influences it, but is both cause and effect of it. They are interopposed, not in the sense that are they enemies, but that they each rely on each other as day follows night. They can be seen as friends, divided by a space which affords life through time. They are interdependent: as with teams in a tug of war, there is no satisfaction unless closely matched. They support each other, but they also consume each other, creating then destroying in turn. Losing yin means gaining yang; but yang needs yin for its means of life, so searches for it — as a mother seeks out her lost child, as a man needs a woman, as a childless woman pines for life within her; each finding purpose in the other.

They also transform each other, as cool air on a fevered brow can eventually chill; we shiver to warm ourselves. Thus at certain stages and under certain conditions depending on time, each turns into its opposite. Quiescence follows motion. Degeneration is due to transformation; we degenerate food as we digest it, enriching ourselves with the nutrients.

It may be added that these four great principles, interopposition, interdependence, mutual consuming and mutual transformation, predispose inherent instability, without which there could be no change. Nothing stays as it is, and there is no perfect balance, although that mean point is what we constantly strive for. Health means a flux round a certain point of reference. If we over-use our energy we grow tired and need rest. Rest too much and we grow bored and long for excitement. Skill in life is acquired by recognizing our limits and turning back before we reach them. The old adage to eat well, but always to leave room for more if long life be desired, illustrates this. These then are the similarities between the two systems, summed up in the image of a hill on which the sun shines: one side is sunny, the other dark. At different times we need the warmth and light, the cool and dark. Without the sun, or without the hill, we could not exist: man stands in the space between Heaven and Earth; 'One yin and one yang are the Tao'.

In traditional Chinese medicine, yin (in relation to yang) is structural potential whereas yang (in relation to yin) is configurative force. So yin is our building, the body; yang is the force within that vivifies and gives shape to our life. Yang moves and warms; yin is the matter moved, and it retards and cools. Someone very yin in condition lacks yang, so is cold and sluggish; if too yang, he is hot and over-reacts. Yang (heat) rises; yin (cold) descends.

Compare these with macrobiotics where yin is centrifugal and expansive, yang is centripetal and contractive. The disparity is clearest if yin (Chinese) cold, inertia, matter, heavy, winter is compared with yin (Macrobiotic) cold, expansion light, growth, i.e. summer. In Chinese thought, yin is not so much a force in itself as that which yang (the force) acts upon, whereas in Macrobiotics yin is a force of expansion opposed to the yang force of contraction. In Chinese thought a food having yin associations would cool and retard, which agrees with Macrobiotics, and an individual who lacked yang would often have a large flabby tongue — demonstrating the Macrobiotic yin tendency or expansion. Chinese yang warms, so eventually dries out, which causes contraction as under Macrobiotic yang. Chinese yin also contracts if there is no yang to warm and expand it, although this is because in cold exterior conditions Chinese yang rises to the surface and contracts, preserving the blood (yin) inside. So the two uses of yin and yang are not exactly opposite, but differ in emphasis, and those who approach Chinese medicine from a Macrobiotic background would do well to regard their knowledge of it as to be used with caution until they are familiar with the Chinese approach. Macrobiotics and Chinese philosophies used together will initially confuse. Later, they can only enrich one another.

Henceforth, when speaking of yin or yang it will be the Chinese model that is meant.

Yin and Yang in Traditional Chinese Medicine

In relation to yang, the mover, yin is that which is moved. When we cut a finger, blood spurts out; the energy which makes it spurt is yang, and the blood that we see is yin. But blood itself has, in relation to the bones and other fixed structures, a yang role in that it moves nourishment to them, warms and activates them. So bones are in at least one sense more yin than blood. They are more static, more structural. In terms of personality, yin is less active, steadier, slower; yang is more excitable, less stable, more energetic. Yin needs yang to warm and vivify it. Yang needs yin to centre and earth it.

Someone very yang is like a small child, running about fast, making lots of noise, getting all the attention and using up energy very fast. The child is also growing fast so eats often and plenty. As we grow older, we grow larger and slower, we use up our energy more slowly and although we have more resources to draw upon, it takes longer to recuperate if we are exhausted, whereas a child quickly exhausts itself but recovers fast. Imagine a small child who sees snow for the first time. He cannot wait to build a snowman and throw a snowball, all the while laughing hysterically. He rapidly warms up and sheds his warm clothes. Suddenly his hands are blue, he is crying and shivering, and he wants his mother's warmth and love. Like a hot air balloon gone cold, he crashes to the earth: but give him a warm drink, the care he needs and a quick doze, and shortly he is up and off again.

We have here a perfect picture of a bundle of yang with a small body (not much yin) that exhausts its yang very fast, and lacks either the experience (a yin word) to know its limitations or the energetic resources to draw upon to persevere for longer. The body (yin) is too small to balance all that childish glee and enthusiasm (yang) and the wise parent watches carefully to preserve the child from harm. In this instance the parent fulfils the child's need for yin. As the child grows older and bigger, dependence on its parents is reduced, and if all goes well, soon after adolescence it may be ready to explore, having developed its own steady centre, helped and taught by its elders.

The image of the small child is also useful because it shows the terrible danger of harming the yin in early childhood by making too many demands on it. The child's growth will then be unbalanced or stunted, and he may all his life unconsciously be looking for a replacement for that stunted or impoverished yin, by working in an environment such as a large factory or government department; or through ill health, depending on others for food and support. If he has been overmothered at too early a stage, he may never overcome that sense of loss, or grief, when perhaps a younger sibling arrived, and will expect to be mothered and protected all his life, placing impossible demands upon partners and friends, and wreaking vengeance for shattered dreams. In this case, the yin was adequately nourished but the yang could not grow properly, so the child expects the partner in adult life to provide excitement and interest and warmth while he plays the big baby who always needs suckling and cuddling.

Yin then is the structure; it has weight and substance; it descends, it absorbs, it is conservative; it has its being in repose and quiet rest; it is static, inactive, quiescent, passive. But it is also sustaining, preserving and nourishing. It confirms, condenses things into matter, completes and perfects them. In itself it is definite and determinate, but it lacks organization.

In terms of energy, it sinks, is sunken or prolapsed, depressed, slow. It makes energy go down and it holds it down.

In terms of the body, it relates to the inside, the internal and deep meridian pathways of energy, the five zang (liver, heart, spleen, lungs, kidneys) the lower part, especially the abdomen, the front (the part we show people when we are receptive to them and we want to hear them), the bones and fluids including blood, the muscles and the flesh. It represents the parasympathetic system in that it slows and rests and recuperates.

In terms of times and seasons, it is the afternoon and night, autumn and winter, when we stay inside more, when some species hibernate. In winter, we should rest more, eat well, replenish our reserves, keep warm, undertake less new, exciting or tiring projects. It is a time better for defence than offence; a time suited more to contemplation, meditation; ideally not a good time for extended energetic actions beyond those we need to preserve, sustain and warm us. A time when we draw on the food we have stored from the summer harvests so that we may be strong again in the spring. The autumn and winter are the times of completion of the year.

As we grow older, our bodies grow slower, more static, we rest more, we lack the spontaneity of youth. Our bodies grow more yin because their yang is used up. If we have spent our lives well, then we have refined our souls, which become our yang aspect, separating from the body (yin) when we die. The soul then becomes the yang aspect, the child, and the body is absorbed into the earth to nourish the Tao in its own way. We say 'the autumn of our lives' to mean that time towards old age when we can enjoy the fruits of our lives and enjoy ourselves in harmless but elevating pastimes that enrich our souls. All too rare are those amongst the old who though old in body are young in spirit, can accept reverses with equanimity and insight, who give back the fruits of their years through compassion, inspiration and teaching, yet do not weary themselves.

In terms of pathology, yin states occur when there is insufficient yang, so the pulse is slow, weak, intermittent, short or deep. There is slowness, coldness, torpor, confusion, weakness, dullness; things don't move properly, they stagnate and we feel heavy, whether in spirit or in body. Pain is dull and chronic.

If yin is that which is moved, but nourishes and cools, YANG is that which moves, needs feeding, and warms. Its nature is to put things into motion, to set them loose, to sublimate, to expand and make active. It brings about change and transforms, it raises things up, it is aggressive and attacks, demands. It is centrifugal and brings rubbish to the surface and expels it. It disperses; it burns. It defends, organizes and holds yin in place.

Its dynamic energy is that of rising, of floating. It sends energy up. It is hot and dry, light, bright and windy. It is daytime when we are most active; spring and summer.

In the body, it is the outside defence, our skin, the upper part, the back, the five fu (Stomach, Small Intestine, Colon, Bladder and Gall Bladder). If someone punches us we tend to protect ourselves with our arms (upper limbs) and to turn sideways or back on, so as to protect our soft abdomen. (If we want to cut somebody off, we turn our back on them, slam the door in their faces, shout at them; all yang activities.) In the meridians of energy, it is the superficial pathways, the tendon and muscular meridians and the Lo (connecting) meridians. It represents the sympathetic nervous system which responds energetically and actively for aggression, escape or defence.

Yang is that which excites and stimulates; we want to dance and move. Many patients who come from the worlds of dance, drama, film production, advertising and cut-throat competition have to be yang to survive. They must always be cheerful, happy, confident, inspired, spontaneous, full of energy, competitive, active. If their work fails to inspire them sufficiently, they grow tired and depressed and take stimulants or energizers to force themselves to peak activity. They tend to be active, impatient and restless. They eat too little or, just as bad, too much, and will not rest. If this continues for too long, they use up their reserves (yin) and cannot rest; they are unrefreshed by their sleep, or sleep badly. They become nervous, irritable and complaining. They then need tranquillizers and relaxants. These drugs upset their yin still more and they begin to fluctuate between wild optimism and exhausted depression. The drugs (stimulants or tranquillizers) substitute for and frequently inhibit the body's own yin and yang, its immunological and defensive recuperative capability. People on heavy drugs are hard to treat, because the drugs actually work against the very energies that need to be strengthened. Patients often fear to reduce their drugs, and the therapist may have to proceed very cautiously as results are unpredictable — at the same time the patient often needs great reassurance yet complains vociferously if results are not immediate! All of this points to a severely damaged yin and a yang that is out of control — somewhat like the small child.

So in terms of pathology, yang states occur when there is either excess yang or insufficient yin: the pulse is fast, superficial, often full or large. Patients over-react, they act too fast, they shout, are angry or hysterical; pain is acute and sudden, of recent onset, and things move too fast and lack control (such as sudden flushes). Patients are restless and demanding, always trying to organize or reorganize things anew. They are very defensive, and can be very destructive. They tend to suffer from problems from chest level upwards (yin suffers from chest level downwards), such as tension in the shoulders and headaches.

Summary of yin and yang qi functions

Yin qi	Yang qi
Cools	Warms
Provides rest, inactivity	Moves, transforms, disperses
Nourishes	Protects
Holds down	Holds up

Compare the above with the tendencies of yin in the absence of yang, and yang in the absence of yin, as follows:

Yin tendency	Yang tendency
Concentrates	Expands
Goes down, descends	Goes up, ascends
Goes inside	Goes outside
Goes in front	Goes to the back
Goes to the right	Goes to the left
Happens during rest, or at night	Happens during activity, or in the day

So (in theory!) someone with a pain in their right abdomen which is worse at night is likely to be suffering from stagnation there due to a deficiency of yang. A problem that occurs in hot weather on the outside and is worse during the day might be due to deficient yin. The former patient is probably lacking in energy, is dispirited, slow to react and somewhat lethargic; the latter is more active and energetic.

In general, symptoms on the outside, or those that are due to some kind of hyperactivity or heat, are yang type, whereas symptoms occuring inside, due to stagnation or cold, are yin type.

Symptoms in Disease

Yin symptoms (= False yin)	Yang symptoms (= Full yang)
Drowsy, quiet, tired	Restless, active
Slow, weak	Rapid movement
Lies down curled up	Lies extended, stretched out
Lies face down	Lies face up
Chilly type, better for heat	Hot type, better in cool conditions
Voice is low and weak	Voice is coarse, rough, loud
Speaks little	Talkative
Breathing is shallow	Breathing is full
Short of breath	
Acid smell	Putrid smell
Facial pallor	Flushed complexion
Pain is dull; aches	Pain is sharp
Likes touch, pressure, warmth	Dislikes touch and heat

Appetite reduced	Dry mouth, thirst
Urine clear, copious	*Urine* dark and scanty
Menses pale and scanty	*Menses* early, profuse, thick
If *constipated*, stagnation is due to lack of peristalsis	*Constipation* characterized by heat and dryness: discomfort
Underreacts	*Overreacts*
Confused, can't decide	Individualistic, orders people around
Muddled: no plans	Irritable, tense, violent
Depressed, weepy	Accident prone
Seeks comfort and advice	
Timid: *slow* response	Aggressive, *quick* response
Can't remember	
Tongue: pale, moist, puffy	*Tongue:* red/scarlet
Moss: thin and white	*Moss:* thick and yellow
Pulse: thin, empty, weak	*Pulse:* full, rapid, wiry, slippery, strong
Low Blood Pressure	High Blood Pressure

It will be noticed that on the left are symptoms caused by a deficiency of yang; on the right are symptoms caused by excess yang. We should expect the yin symptoms to occur after a long exhausting illness; the yang symptoms are much more acute, and whilst they may be more immediately unpleasant and dangerous, they rarely continue for long. Yin symptoms — meaning yang deficiency — may be less dangerous, but they take longer to cure. In an old person they may be impossible to cure.

Strictly speaking, the yin symptoms above should be called 'False yin' symptoms, because they are not due to excess yin but are due to deficient yang.

There are also symptoms known as 'False yang', caused by deficient yin: these are common, and important.

False yang symptoms
(due to deficiency of yin)
Debility; uneasy, nervous movement, weak and rapid
Irritability without force or persistence
Reacts quickly but weakly
Feels hot, but cools rapidly, or averse to uncovering
Emaciation
Insomnia: cannot sleep deeply; frequent wakings

Sweats at night not due to heat of room or bed

Fever or feeling of heat on torso or head, particularly noticeable in the afternoon, often accompanied by thirst at that time

Cheeks: flush over the cheek bones

Throat dry: drinking doesn't really quench thirst. Keeps needing to sip cool water

Palms and soles feel burning, though may not be especially hot to the touch

Constipation: stools are dry. Urine is dark, scanty

Eyes have spots in them: may tire easily

Menses: scanty, late, absent, ache

Tongue: reddish

Pulse: fast but thin.

False yang occurs after a period of chronic disease, too much work or sex, though it can be due to constitutional or dietary deficiences. Compare it with Kidney yin deficiency (q.v.).

The remaining factor is full yin, caused by invasion of the body by overwhelming yin, i.e. cold. The cold causes stagnation, so pressure worsens pain, which is better for warmth.

Full yin symptoms

Internal temperature drops

Capillaries may turn blue

Feels cold: likes warmth

Body feels heavy: movement is slow, clumsy and laborious

Sleepy, anxious

Menses: painful, stabbing pains; delayed

Tongue: moist and pale, can even look blue

Moss: pale

Pulse: forceful but slow.

These four states — full or excess yang, deficient yang (false yin), deficiency of yin (false yang), and full or excess yin are basic states, although there are usually other complicating factors. But they are enough to begin to consider how we may expect planets to indicate changes in health.

8.

YIN, YANG, BLOOD AND QI

Yin type planets		Yang type planets	
	Sun, Moon and Ancient Planets		
☽	Moon	☉	Sun
♀	Venus	♂	Mars
♄	Saturn	♃	Jupiter
☿	Mercury	☿	Mercury

Extra-Saturnian Planets

♇	Pluto	♆	Neptune	♅	Uranus

Sun, Moon and Ancient Planets

If the discussion of the four-phase diagram has been followed, then it should not be difficult to see why Venus, Saturn and Mercury are yin, nor why Mars, Jupiter and Mercury are yang. Mercury appears twice, representing dual aspects. The Sun is the originator of all yang, but we should be wary of assuming that it has no yin, as it is the most stabilizing, centralizing, integrating force of all. Nevertheless, few astrologers would dispute that it is predominantly yang.

The question of the Moon is more complicated. In astrological tradition it appears as receptive and habitual, giving rhythmic movement to life. This movement may seem to point to a strong yang component — which it has. However, this rhythm preserves the status quo of life — e.g. steady heartbeat, respiration while asleep, menstrual cycle, intestinal peristalsis, movement of lymph. The reason is to nourish and preserve, to recover energy — all activities to maintain the body in ordinary working order. In a wider context, it covers all everyday activities that give the means to preserve health, including job, family and home.

In so far as these everyday activities are consciously aimed at preserving the health of the body, the family and the community, they are lunar in essence. The same goes for activities that have become habitual and are done without conscious thought, because such activities are built in to the ordinary living pattern, so maintain the status quo, whether or not they are health-giving. Our lives are run 99 per cent of the time on habit. We don't often need to think about how to get to work, yet we do it every day: put hand on railing, set foot on stair, sit on seat, place fingers on gearstick. When we arrive at work: open door, walk to workplace, set up tools, smile at neighbours, work mechanisms, stop for rest, continue routine, pick up wages, go home. Personal habits are the same: frown, pick nose, scratch ear, get drunk, keep money in purse, smoke, handkerchief in left pocket, door key round neck, snore when asleep; morning exercise, jog, swim, stand on head; food - averse to vegetables, like fat, want more whisky/beer/wine/water.

Most such habits once needed conscious effort to begin. They are very hard to alter, as smokers know to their cost! All such habits give order to our lives: if you smoke, just try using different fingers to hold the cigarette, and see how long it takes to feel comfortable! Changes to our system of living can be very threatening. The strength of our yang planets determines how we react, how willingly we set out to defend ourselves. What we are defending is represented mainly by the Moon, be it our family, our union, our standard of living, the colour of our bedsocks or our country.

The predominant force that initiates such habits is represented by the Sun, which gives us the seasons, and our New Year resolutions. When we move house or change jobs from clearly conscious motives, we operate on our Sun level. On starting the new job we have to choose new habits, both to get to work and to do the job. Strongly developed Sun types need less help than the rest of us Moon types.

It is a mistake to assume that all lunar activities are unconscious, all solar activities conscious. This is a dualist approach, and traditional Chinese medicine is not dualistic, though for convenience yin and yang are chosen to represent two aspects of life.

It has been fashionable to argue that a dominant rational discriminating attitude is male and that all thought forms or processes which have been repressed or neglected by this are female. But it can be as habitual to think rationally and analytically as to think intuitively and qualitatively. As Jung has suggested, the opposite way of thinking may be quite difficult, whichever is one's sex.

Unfortunately the Moon has been associated with femininity, the

Sun with masculinity. If traditional Chinese medicine is any guide, the Moon should be associated with those activities that further the orderly continuation of the body in a harmonious family, community or national background, whereas the Sun relates to those forces that shape the individual, that incline him to be different, to follow his own destiny. Lunar forces make us all the same. The Sun makes us different. Statistics are based on observations of lunar predisposition; they cannot account for solar eccentricity.

Lunar traits	*Solar traits*
Confirming	Beginning
Sustaining	Setting loose
Condensing	Dispersing
Reposing	Transforming
Awaiting	Developing
Receptive	Outgoing
Enduring	Sense of self
Never breaking	Independence
Yielding	Ability to focus
Listening	
Accepting	
Waiting	
Trusting	

These lists are a risk! A strongly placed Moon in Cancer, without challenging aspects from yang planets, may well give the individual some of the lunar traits listed. But if placed in Aries (say) or conjunct Mars, then such traits would be much less obvious and the individual might need to cultivate gentler lunar traits to maintain health.

Equally, life becomes dull without change, and the Sun urges us to move on, to explore, to challenge. It is the Sun that heats the air to provide the wind that blows away cobwebs. It is the Sun whose light is reflected by the Moon. Why do we blame the Moon for the acknowledged changes in unstable individuals or groups that occur at New or Full Moon? What we are witnessing are not lunar traits, but solar traits occurring in people whose lunar ways are not strong enough to preserve them from accident. And lunatics are individuals whose solar forces cannot be contained.

We can now see why problems such as insanity and epilepsy are astrologically closely related and why, in terms of traditional Chinese medicine, they occur. Both can involve any of the planets, Sun and

Moon, but in traditional Western astrology Mercury and the Moon are nearly always important, often in aspect to the Ascendant, the gateway to the personality.

The Moon relates to all the zangfu, but notably to the Earth phase, governed by Saturn. Many of its traits listed above are yin traits, and come close to the functions of Earth, nourishing and preserving the vehicle in which the life cycle of four phases occurs. This Earth is the stuff in which qi manifests. The Water — Mercury phase describes the quiescent and waiting aspects of yin. Together, Water and Earth represent yin most clearly. When these energies are unable to contain the extrovert forces of yang, life is threatened and mania or epilepsy can occur. (To a lesser extent, the same occurs when the temper is lost: we see red; our blood boils; we lose control. Drugs and alcohol can have a similar effect, weakening the grasp between yin and yang, between body and spirit.)

There are many kinds of insanity. Not all are due to this split between yin and yang. The confusion and apathy of suicidal melancholia suggests a yang that is exhausted and cannot function through a relatively overwhelming yin — and a yin that is unclean and fogbound. Traditional Chinese medicine has an explanation for this, separately discussed under 'damp'.

Blood and Qi

These are aspects of yin and yang; but whereas yin and yang are abstract, Blood and qi are much easier to appreciate. Qi, vitality, carries its energy to all parts through the medium of the Blood.

Blood	Qi
A foundation for qi to organize	Source of movement
Cools and moistens	Warms and dries
Nourishes and calms	Protects
Balances excess qi	Transforms
Harmonizes and rests	Maintains things in place
Vehicle for *hun* — soul — (housed by Liver)	

Some of this needs explanation. Qi and movement go together. It is misleading to say that qi creates or causes movement, because qi and movement are inseparable, whether the movement be one of blood circulation, growth, bodily exertion (running, swimming, talking) or mental activity.

The initial foundation or substratum in which qi manifests is Blood. 'Blood' includes the red liquid that we carry in our veins, but is also said to flow along the meridians, which are contacted with acupuncture needles. Blood, in traditional Chinese medicine, is actually a form of liquid qi; nearly everything discussed in this book is considered as a manifestation of qi, and Blood is one of the more yin kinds of qi. (There is another important group of fluids known as 'jinye', which includes tears and saliva. For present purposes these are discussed as though they were part of Blood.)

The cooling, moistening, balancing function of Blood acts as an anchor and balance for qi. If we are hot, then there is insufficient Blood to cool us.

The protecting role of qi works by guarding the Blood and by maintaining fluids where they belong. Sudden haemorrhage, incontinence, spontaneous sweating and dribbling from the mouth are examples of a failure by qi to hold things in place. The transforming aspect of qi is seen in the process of digestion, where food is turned into energy which can be used for action.

While there is life, Blood and qi are inseparable: hence the phrase, 'Qi is the leader of Blood, Blood the attachment for qi.'

The importance of the theory of the Blood and qi in traditional Chinese medicine can hardly be emphasized too strongly. Blood and qi constitute the fundamental base for physiological functioning. Blood is formed from food essence, and its nutrient substance is transported to all of the zangfu organs, the skin, hair, muscles, tendons, bones, meridians and subsidiary vessels. Formation of Blood relies on the normal functional activities of the zangfu, especially Spleen (Spleen produces Blood), Heart (Heart dominates Blood), and Lung (Lung dominates qi).

'Qi is the commander of Blood: the free flow of qi carries a smooth flow of Blood. Stopping qi movement stops Blood flow. If qi is invaded by cold (cold qi), this causes coagulation of Blood.' (Yang Shiyin).

So pathological changes in Blood follow changes in qi. Qi warms, so patients with deficient qi are averse to cold. Blood moistens and nourishes the body; if Blood is deficient there is usually a dry skin. But Blood flow and circulation depends on the function of qi in warming the body.

'Blood and qi are fond of warmth, and averse to cold.' (Neijing).

Invasion of cold causes obstruction of qi and Blood, which can be resolved by warming up.

Many diseases are complicated, but most relate to qi and Blood. Equally, disharmony of qi and Blood causes many diseases. Because they are so closely related, disease in qi will affect Blood and vice versa. So deficient qi leads to deficient Blood; and deficiency of Blood leads to deficient qi. It has been said that 'when qi and Blood are in balance, people are healthy, so live long lives'. Also: 'The secret of treating disease is to have a clear understanding of qi and Blood. No matter what kind of disease, balance between qi and Blood should be given priority.'

There are many examples of disharmonies between qi and Blood. Common are:

1. Weak qi leads to deficient Blood.
2. Deficient Blood leads to deficient qi.
3. Deficient qi leads to congealed Blood.
4. Stagnant qi leads to congealed Blood.
5. Irregular flow of Blood due to adverse qi circulation.
6. Qi fails to control Blood, leading to exhaustion of Blood and qi.

1. Weak qi leads to Blood deficiency

Here we see clear signs of anaemia as well as qi deficiency.

Symptoms might be: sallow complexion, stuffy chest, poor appetite, abdominal distension after a meal, loose stools and general lassitude. Assuming no history of haemorrhage, these symptoms indicate weak Spleen qi being unable to produce good qi and Blood, the usual causes being irregularities in diet, over-exertion and chronic disease.

2. Blood deficiency causes qi deficiency

This is often seen in chronic haemorrhagic disease, such as is due to prolonged intestinal bleeding, or dysfunctional bleeding from the uterus. Haemorrhage being the main symptom leads first to Blood deficiency, then qi deficiency, characterized by lassitude. This state also occurs in cases of acute massive bleeding, when priority must be to stop the bleeding, and if necessary give fresh blood.

3. Qi deficiency leads to congealed Blood

This often occurs after long illness, or after apoplexy. The clinical manifestation is 'congealed' Blood; numbness of local skin; no sensation. Local pain, sometimes purpura. Tongue goes purple; red marks on the face.

Another example might be epigastric pain of many years duration, e.g. gastritis. Here pain is often better for pressure, and we should expect to find other signs of qi deficiency, such as a weak voice, pale complexion, pale tongue with toothmarks round it. The symptoms of congealed Blood are pain that remains fixed in a given locality. Pulse is often uneven, indicating uneven blood flow. There might also be poor appetite and some regurgitation.

Here deficient qi has lost the ability to promote smooth blood flow. Treatment aims to tonify qi and warm yang.

4. Stagnant qi leads to congealed Blood

Stagnant qi nearly always means Liver qi stagnation. (The other main cause is Cold, which contracts and tightens.) Here the congealed Blood occurs mainly in the abdomen, the area partly 'ruled' by the Liver, and symptoms such as dysmenorrhoea and epigastric pain, of a cramping, distending nature, are common. (Stagnation due to cold causes a pain that is stabbing and acute.) Involvements of Liver suggests mental depression as a concomitant symptom.

5. Irregular flow of Blood due to adverse qi circulation

Adverse qi circulation means that the zangfu organs have lost their normal functional activities, so instead of sending yin upwards (to moisten, nourish and cool) and yang downwards (to warm and move), yin descends and yang ascends. This is a broad picture, only partly related to the direction of flow of qi in the meridians (yin meridians flow upwards; yang meridians flow downwards), because each zangfu organ has its own action, which if qi circulates in an adverse direction, will go in the wrong direction. Both ascending and descending adverse qi can lead to haemorrhage, as for example:

Adverse qi in Liver and Stomach	— haemetemesis
Adverse qi in Lung	— haemoptysis
Upward attack of qi to brain	— syncope, cerebral haemorrhage
Adverse descending of Spleen qi	— blood in stools and dysfunctional uterine bleeding

Note that Liver qi should ascend (among other actions): here we mean adverse excessive ascending Liver qi. Stomach qi should descend: if it ascends, we get nausea, vomiting and potentially, as above, haematemesis. Upward attack of qi to the brain can occur in sudden fainting, perhaps due to emotional causes. Dysfunctional uterine bleeding has other causes than the above.

6. Qi fails to control Blood, causing exhaustion of Blood, followed by exhaustion of qi

By failure to control blood, we mean dysfunction of Spleen in controlling blood i.e. deficient Spleen qi. Here the failure leads to leakage, so there are signs of haemorrhage (uterine, purpura, etc.) accompanied by signs of weak Spleen qi. It occurs in such cases as massive uterine bleeding, or severe vomiting of blood. Owing to the severity, we find pallor, cold limbs, profuse sweating, low voice and incoherent or interrupted speech patterns. In severe cases this is followed by syncope. These signs are due to exhausted qi caused by Blood exhaustion.

As can be seen, the above occur in more or less increasing order of severity. For such a large and important subject, this is the briefest of introductions. From an astrological point of view, it is interesting to consider the transits and progressions of, in particular, Sun and Moon in these more serious cases. In the less obvious, but commoner, cases such as anaemia due to weak qi, the aspects to natal position of Sun and Moon are particularly important. Carter's *The Astrological Aspects* contains a masterly account of the effect of Sun-Moon aspects, very relevant in consideration of the chart discussed later in this chapter.

Perusal of what he has to say about Sun-Moon inharmonious aspects points to a lack of flow between different sides of the personality. The term 'lack of flow' suggests tendency to stagnant Liver qi, with all that implies in terms of emotional disorder. Liver stores the Blood in traditional Chinese medicine, and we might therefore expect to find sporadic insomnia, or sleep that is not refreshing. There might also be cramps and spasms — physical reflections of the native's 'brusque and rude manners', and an unreliable gastro-intestinal tract to match the 'changeable demeanour'.

In terms of the effect on qi and Blood, we expect someone who works in bouts, with exhausting enthusiasm. He takes on too much, then overworks, causing qi deficiency, with uncertainty of aim, tiredness, poor decision-making ability and chilliness. This leads to a sallow complexion, a lack of calmness and a search for identity, for a home, for harmony. Because qi lacks a home in Blood, he searches always for new philosophies and new cures, growing ever more tired, but always looking for that final solution, that famous guru, a magnetic strength that will heal him of all his woes. He has lost qi, he has weakened his Blood, so yang and yin are less strongly connected, and he is unable calmly and with consideration to make mature relationships.

What advice can one give someone with this type of problem? Traditional Chinese medicine points to both Blood and qi being at fault, but priority must be given to nourishing qi. So rest, calmness and avoidance of worrying situations are prerequisite — rest, because this conserves qi; calmness and avoidance of worry because they are important for allowing Spleen qi to learn again to transform food into Blood and qi. (Note that 'obsession' and 'over-thinking' are both bad for Spleen.) The patient should keep warm, take gentle exercise and on no account exhaust himself either physically or emotionally. He should reduce sexual exertion, sleep a lot, and allow himself to recoup. Treatment might be nutritional, autogenic or phsycho-therapeutic as well as via herbs. Acupuncture is of course excellent for rebalancing many such disharmonies. Holidays that are exciting, hazardous, too hot or too cold, exhausting or with indigestible diets are not conducive! Is it surprising that many of these individuals lead a somewhat 'withdrawn' life?

But how do they guard against such exhaustion? The Tao Te Ching suggests that:

> In managing life, the best advice is to be sparing.
> To be sparing is to forestall.
> To forestall is to be prepared and strengthened.
> To be prepared and strengthened is to be ever successful.
> To be ever successful is to know no bounds.

In this advice we see the emphasis on conserving qi, on protecting and strengthening the Blood, so that from that strong lunar centre, our solar energy can irradiate life.

Extra-Saturnian Planets

The ancient Chinese were not aware of Uranus (♅), Neptune (♆) and Pluto (♇). The following is one possible allocation of their energies.

Pluto and Kidney qi

Variously associated with transformation, death, resurrection, deep traumatic episodes in personality developments when an old structure has to be destroyed to make way for the new, Pluto is a necessary part of growth; growth that forces its way through an established, stultified status quo. The charismatic magnetism Plutonians display comes from their ability to break free of stasis, not by madcap revolution but by wielding great power behind the scenes. Pluto is associated with the release of tension in sexual orgasm, the 'little death'. Its power for transformation is often apparent in the charts of those who, having undergone some form of transformation themselves, are able to assist others likewise (e.g. in the charts of therapists, be they healers or acupuncturists, psychologists or homoeopaths). One thing is certain: these individuals may employ useful techniques but they are not technicians; they never cease to search for deeper meaning, knowledge and power in their lives. Life for them is impossible unless there is some deep hidden fire pushing them towards greater awareness, challenging the established order of their lives.

Pluto is closely related to Scorpio, which shares the same reserves of power, for good or ill. These energies if used for personal benefit will eventually bring harm and evil. Mars has self-assertive power, but it is not hidden, and Venus responds to it with open enmity or co-operation (via ♎, opposite ♈, ruled by ♀) or material well-being and nourishment (via ♉). But Pluto's power used selfishly tries to control its environment, to bind all others into its forcefield, and the effects, instead of being transformative from lower to higher levels of awareness, are destructive of life.

Its power to transform through a process akin to dying gives Pluto a strong relationship with the Water phase. Perhaps we may adduce an analogy with its astronomical distance from the Sun: if Sun and Fire phases are related, then Pluto, furthest from the Sun, relates to Water phase, that phase in which life appears least active, but in which the miracle of creation seeks germination. There is a corollary with the genetic code which in traditional Chinese medicine is associated with Kidney energy. Kidney qi includes the growth patterns of the individual, and Pluto's power certainly partakes of these. In being magnetized into the Plutonian's forcefield, are we not being forced into the pattern of his genetic code? Is he not seeking to shape us in his mould, rather than trying to break out of that mould himself? This is yin coercing yang, rather than allowing yang to change it; it is an attempt to prevent change except according to its own wishes. The pattern promised may be exciting, but it is not *our* pattern.

Those of Plutonian inclination but less powerful over others will look to drugs and sexual activities. Kidney qi, it has already been explained, is closely connected with the sexual power and its abuse. Drugs are another way of achieving the energy that good Kidney qi disposes — albeit at the longer-term expense of the Kidneys. Kundalini energy rises up the spine to the head, and with suitable disciplines is a renewing and transforming energy. Its path and source follow closely the energetic arrangement of Kidney qi, whose yin aspects moisten the spinal cord and brain, the 'Sea of Marrow'. When not so disciplined, could not the same force be partly responsible for some epileptic states, especially those occurring at night or in sleep, the yin period of the day?

In Western astrology, Pluto is closely related to the process of elimination. Kidney qi covers many aspects of fluid metabolism and excretion, and accords with Pluto's action of bringing outworn processes to the surface, of purging old complexes, patterns and tensions.

(But all phases partake of the nature of their opposite, especially when they malfunction, and Pluto may be partly representative of the searching intuitive percipience of those who heal through the *Fiery* power of their soul and of the energies pouring through them. None of the extra-Saturnian planets, and certainly not Pluto, can be entirely forced into one energy system.)

Finally, it seems to me that Pluto partakes more of the nature of Kidney yang.

Uranus and Liver qi

Whereas Pluto seems to give a completely new departure of life through a process of internal elimination, Uranus is much more obvious. Pluto's effect can take ages to work out. Uranus is sudden, dramatic, forceful. It gives originality, independent self-expression, and a desire to break away from tradition. The mind is not transformed, as with Pluto, but organizes life on new lines. It is well to be clear about this difference. Change in a Uranian's life may be sudden, unplanned, and disruptive, but the personality coheres. In a Plutonian's life-change, there is an actual alteration in personality, usually painful, due to destruction of old and creation of new patterns of being. The Uranian may change his mind — he not infrequently does, and pursues his new belief with maniacal enthusiasm — but he does not lose his identity in the process. At best he entertains new ideas objectively and detachedly, hence the relationship between Uranus and Aquarius.

When things flow smoothly for the Uranian, he can be a force for reform, with an inventive unconventionality and independence that can amount to genius. When the Uranian spirit is unable so to function, we get impatience, ruthlessness, fanaticism and irresponsibility. All these lead to tension and stagnation of Liver qi. So although it would be a mistake to say that Uranus rules Liver, it is nevertheless strongly implicated. If Jupiter broadens our horizons,

Uranus stretches and twists more new opportunities to its own ends. Obstructed, it revels in eccentric fury — definitely a very 'Wood' type phenomenon!

Uranus has been said to operate on a higher plane or octave but with the same kind of action as Mercury. If Mercury gives intelligence, Uranus gives genius. The four-phase diagram shows how, if for the moment Uranus is given to Wood, the energies of both Jupiter and Uranus receive nourishment from the energy of Water phase. If Water is weak (i.e. in a chart, if ♇ or ☿ lack strength) then there will be no sure foundation for the experimentation of Wood (♃ and ♅); so the individual's ideas will be half-baked. Power in ☿ and ♇ gives the strength to think things through and to persevere; the tree's roots are then deeply laid, and no storm can overturn it. Similarly, the spasms and nervous excitability of the wayward Uranian are held firmly by the strength of Water. So, lacking Water's control, we may find Wood energy ascending too freely, leading to hysteria, nervous excitability, palpitations and breakdown. There may be cramps, spasms, tremors, tics and even paralysis.

Neptune

Neptunians are somewhat indiscriminate, and find it hard to say no. All relationships need an element of Neptune, first through the power of suggestion and dream to entice each into the other's arms, and then by blurring boundaries so that neither feels too threatened. Neptunians lack a clear sense of their own identity: either they dissipate their energy or they compensate by copying another or moulding themselves to the pattern of a firm leader of faith. There is nearly always a strong sense of idealism in their nature, due to uncertainty about the self, the needs of which they find comparatively easy to sacrifice. They give themselves up too easily for others, so dissipate their strength. (Readers without astrological experience should read up Neptune: it has a good side too!)

From this we can see that they are susceptible to qi deficiency: it seems to pour out of them without restraint. But qi deficiency leads to Blood deficiency, which causes an array of symptoms such as anaemia and lassitude, poor tissue formation (e.g. flabbiness), numbness, untraceable pains, loss of identity as in unconsciousness and coma, haemorrhage and leakage of all kinds of fluids, illusions, disorientation and general weakness. They lack resistance to invasion of external pathogenic forces, so easily get infected, and their fluid metabolism is weak. They are usually relaxed or limp.

Clearly these symptoms point at least to Spleen deficiency. Inability to project personality, however, is a Liver weakness. In their loose hold on physical reality there is a schism between yin and yang. Neptunians tend to suffer from strange pains without pathological cause, and it has been surmised that this relates to a close connection with the spinal cord and canal. In traditional Chinese medicine, the spine is closely related to Spleen, the spinal cord and canal to Kidney. So there are arguments for Spleen, Kidney and Liver energies being Neptunian, and indeed each of these yin zangfu organs have meridians that run up the legs and penetrate the abdomen, wherein lies the centre of gravity, the centre of our energy reserves.

At their best, aspects from ♆ enhance intuition, spiritual insight, and psychic sensitivity, frequently turning the individual away from materialism and egocentric desire and sensualism. They produce refined and artistic people who may lack a strong physical and sexual constitution. The inherited constitution comes mainly via Kidney, the growth from Liver, the physical musculature and tissue formation from Spleen.

Max Heindel suggested that ♆ should be considered a higher octave of ☿; others say it is a higher octave of ♀. If the latter, then we should expect ♆ symptoms to be similar to Lung symptoms. Lung deficiency gives, for example, tiredness, a weak voice and susceptibility to infection, and can lead, if due to prolonged grief or worry, to a general deterioration in mind and body. But the indications for association of ♆ and Lung are no stronger than for ♆ and, say, Spleen. However, Lungs are said to dominate qi, and there is no doubt that Neptune weakens qi and the grip it has on Blood. (The eight extra meridians are not discussed in the book, but Neptune has a strong relationship with, for instance, Ren Mo, the master point for which lies on the Lung meridian.) When Neptune's adverse aspects impinge on the individual, he or she finds that there is a blurring between right and wrong, with a tendency to permit outside influences to interfere detrimentally to a continued healthy — that is, whole — state. On the one hand physical instincts and sensations are amplified and exhausted, leading to nervous exhaustion, and the mind reaches into unreal, dreamlike or drug-induced states. On the other hand, there is relaxation of tissues, varying from varicose veins to prolapse, general weakness and flabbiness, neurasthenia, strange sensations without apparent foundation, fluid retention, weakness, confusion and uncertainty. If any emotion is uppermost, it must be that of *fear*; fear especially of loss of control. Fear leads us again to Kidney energy!

Although its effects seem so broad, in a chart one looks mainly at its aspects and position, and it is these which point to specific areas of weakness. Wherever situated, its job seems to be to make connections that undermine the cohesion of the psyche, forcing it to establish broader links with its surroundings, by means either of more enlightened sensitivity or of greater dependence on medical or other outside help. Drugs maintain us in a false state of security; they prevent us from adapting to those forces in our lives that seek to undermine our integrity; they stop us from evolving into greater beings. Neptunian drugs deceive us into thinking we have achieved that strength. When used properly we learn how to maintain our strength in deeper and more refined ways, at the same time benefiting those around us.

In the four phase diagram, Metal represents the refining, discriminating period when we eliminate that which we no longer require. If we are unable to expel the rubbish, or if we absorb influences that confuse and poison us, as when Neptune malfunctions, our energy will deteriorate, and we shall lose our ability to see and choose what is best. Moving from this phase to that of Water, the phase in which we lose ourselves, for example in sleep, a poor Neptunian influence may dissolve our reserves to such an extent that we cannot again recover our identity: we slip quietly away. A growing number of drug addicts lose their grip of reality, denying the rest of us their personalities, until they die, when they leave us (if not before) with guilt and a sense of unresolved dilemma. The death of someone who has clearly perceived who or what he is, and has put his energy towards the improvement of life, leaves a clear space behind, one that is pure and unpoisoned.

Neptune seems to me to relate more to Kidney yin. Unlike Pluto, which forces new life through an old mould, so is more yang, Neptune deals more with a process that refines the old mould, subtly altering its characteristics.

Case 7: Male, 57

Chart 7 is that of someone who suffered from a weak Bladder from an early age — and was ashamed of it. It followed whooping cough, when what was probably no more than a temporary sphincter muscle weakness became chronic after a hospital matron chastized him publicly for his 'lack of self-control' - a terrifying experience. A man of great promise and skill in his work, he was terrified of admitting his weakness to others. This led to a lack of self-confidence in interpersonal relations, and a personality that was withdrawn and dreamy. Pride in his work was considerable, but he was most sensitive

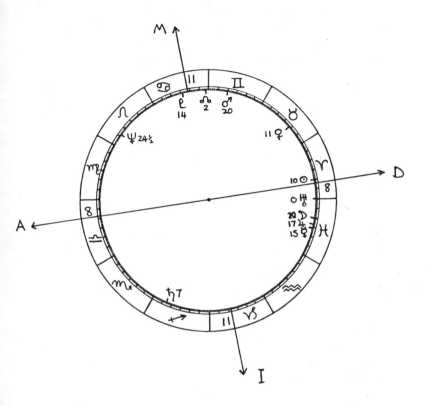

Chart 7. Male, 57.

to criticism. After an accident he had fits and was diagnosed as epileptic, though it is possible that the accident occurred during an epileptic fit; that is, the condition was already present by the age of 23. (He remembered, at about 3 years old, a vivid flash in an accident to his head, and his mother's subsequent hysterical reaction.) He had always suffered from bowel troubles, with years of constipation. He drank heavily from his teens until he was 47, and this no doubt contributed to the failure of his marriage. Stopping alcohol addiction was difficult because it cut him off from his friends. He stopped because after four days of heavy drinking he began to experience strange sensations, culminating in a fit and hospitalization. He says that his personality began to deteriorate from this point onwards, and he lost many of his interests. When he presented himself for treatment he was very depressed and complained of being unable to organize himself or his thinking. He had lack of stamina, poor circulation, varicose veins, poor sleep and no sex drive. He was taking anticonvulsants, which contributed to his mental confusion.

At around 3 years old: PM☌♇, T♅☌☉☌ Desc, P☿☌♃. At around 5 years old: P☉□♇, P☽□☿☽♃, ☌♂, T♃☌♆. (The patient was unable to give precise dates.) The accident at 23 occurred when P☽☍♇, P☿☌☉ ☌ Desc. T♆☍☉, T♅☌M. The drinking bout at 47 seems to have occurred when T♇☌A, T♆☌♄, though he was unsure of the exact date.

The development of his condition in traditional Chinese medicine seems to begin with injury to Kidney qi, leading to weakness of Kidney yang and then to Kidney jing. Epilepsy is associated with weak Kidney yin and Liver yin, which allows Interior Wind to develop, upsetting fluids and sending rebellious qi, or Internal Wind and Phlegm, upwards, disturbing qi in the head. The weak Kidney qi would lead to lack of stamina, poor circulation, poor sleep, urination problems, low sex drive and various other conditions he complained of.

The angular positions of ♇ and ☉ highlight their importance. These are the two extremes of the solar system, and they are square to one another. We might judge ☉ to be weakened by aspects to ♆ and retrograde ♄; ☽ and ☿ to be strengthened by conjunction with ♃, but □♂. The position of ♇ gives him unusual persistence, but is not an enlivening force. It does, however, give him a desire never to be satisfied; to challenge and move on. He is not an ordinary man, and this tendency to be an outsider is supported by retrograde ♄, alone in the first quadrant. Enuresis and weakness of Kidney qi comes partly from ♇, partly ☉⚼♆△♄ (i.e. weakening qi) and partly from the ♂□♃, which affects ☽ and ☿. As Carter points out, the (lunar) early life was subject to impulse and, in this case, accident and injury. But the adult who came for treatment was prudent and controlled, at least in his conscious actions. (The epileptic attacks have recently occurred only at night.) Nevertheless, the powerful solar urge towards self-determination (qi), is weakened by ♆ and — perhaps — too much of a strain for ♇; and the lunar and Mercury fluids (Blood) too easily disturbed by ♂ + ♃, which refuse to allow Kidney energy (☿) to hold firm to what should be held down.

This is therefore a case which can be seen either as a weakness in Kidney qi, or as a disturbance between qi and the fluids. Could one have predicted epilepsy from this chart? Doubtful! But one can probably see the disturbed childhood, unfortunate marriage, lack of self-confidence, fear, and prolonged, though hidden, ill health due weak Kidney qi, etc. Astrologers will note that the position of the

7th house Sun points to unusual importance in the relationship between patient and practitioner.

Yin and Yang Medicine

Orthodox Western medicine is analytical of the body, its parts, blood and pathology. Chinese medicine and health awareness emphasizes the vitality that animates the body. We may describe Western medicine and oriental medicine as 'yin-based' and 'yang-based' respectively.

It has been said that Western medicine has a better grasp of conditions that affect the health arising from a gross change in the physical body, e.g. a tumour or a fracture. Oriental medicine is better where the disease cannot be traced to such a specific change, but is more to do with the energy systems of the body - what drives it.

We see this difference in the approach to contagious disease. The Western approach is to apply treatment to kill the invading organism. The more specific the treatment, the more direct will it be on the 'bug' and the less damaging to the body. The whole tenor of Chinese medicine is to treat the energy situation that allows body and bug to live together. If the body's energy field is friendly to it, the bug will live. But when the environment ceases to be habitable, by a return towards a state called 'health', the bug will lose its foothold. Another way of saying this is that, while ill, the person has lost the key to what it is to be healthy. Treatment should aim to provide that key, as it is implicitly assumed that the energy can, with that help, find its way back to normality, and that the symptoms of the disease are the energy's way of displaying its *dis*-ease.

By recognizing energy as the fundamental cause of health and disease, traditional Chinese medicine draws criticism from those whose understanding encompasses only palpable facts. Qi, prana, orgone, etc., all names for the underlying vitality that gives life, cannot be seen under a microscope. When a man dies, his body remains for autopsy; not so his qi, which has departed.

If we say 'The life has gone out of him,' we recognize this parting of qi and Blood at the moment of death. It is implicit in traditional Chinese medicine that the underlying reality of life manifest is not the body, the vehicle, but the qi within it. Illness is seen as some kind of dysfunction between the life force (= yang, qi) and the body (= yin, Blood). At birth, the life force is very strong and the body a very small anchor for it. Hence, in childhood, the rapid shifts in symptoms of the life force, between sleep, hunger, noise and violent temperature fluctuations, at least in illness. In old age, there remains but little life force to drive the body, which is now large and in poor repair, so symptoms depart much more slowly.

In recognizing two factors in disease, traditional Chinese medicine puts Western medicine at a disadvantage. In recognizing only the yin aspect of disease, Western medicine fails to appreciate the immensely important contribution to the understanding of disease that is made by the emotional, mental and spiritual: yang. And yang has been studied carefully in traditional Chinese medicine for perhaps five millennia.

But this is not to say that traditional Chinese medicine despises yin! The two are equally important. Western medicine has much better resources for studying yin than has traditional Chinese medicine. This goes some way towards explaining why doctors in China have leaped on to the advances of Western medicine with such loud and enthusiastic cries of Oriental glee. Traditional Chinese medicine has very little to lose in embracing Western medical theories and advances. Above all, traditional Chinese medicine is pragmatic: if a theory works, use it. But if it ceases to apply in a particular instance, don't condemn it! Look for another theory to fit the facts, and keep that first theory in reserve; it may be useful another day. No single theory can ever hope to work *all* the time: there is no final 'ring of truth'. But everything works occasionally, and some theories are more serviceable than others — and Western medicine has lots of good ploys.

Practitioners of Western medicine feel threatened by this. For them there is only one ultimately correct answer, and when that is found, all previous answers will be incorrect. Such a solution comes through analysis. To look for it by synthesis, by seeking solutions to problems in the property of a sum that is more than the properties of its parts, is magic — no, worse: lunacy. Yang is magic - either that or placebo!

And that is unfair to traditional Chinese medicine. Yang is no more magic than yin; it is simply a representation of something that has not recently been studied in Western thinking. But in recognizing that placebo exists, Western medicine tacitly assumes that people have an inbuilt force that, given the key — be it a pill, a food or a belief structure — will cure them. Traditional Chinese medicine has studied that force, and it is one of the energies of life that are subsumed in 'qi', an aspect of yang.

9.

ORIGINS OF DISEASE

This chapter is not about the level at which the body's qi erects a barrier — the depth at which disease manifests. Traditional Chinese medicine has plenty to say about this, and an understanding of the various levels at which defences are varied leads to more accurate prognosis of the length and direction of cure, but this must await another book! Equally, this chapter is not about the symptom picture portrayed by a patient who comes for treatment.

It is pertinent to observe that whether or not a practitioner discerns the true cause of a disease, he cannot always expect an easy run if he sets about healing from the inner core of a situation outwards. There may well be aggravations as the invigorated energy forces out the disease. Unless he is invited to work in that way, he may be advised to remove some of the symptoms first — so gaining the patient's trust. Later, if the patient expresses an interest in a more overall cure, he can probe more deeply. It is not always wise to go deeply first, nor are many practitioners trained to do so. The danger of a superficial approach, however, is that in removing some of the symptoms, the practitioner may obscure the overall picture, and may even be guilty of suppressing the disease and weakening the vitality. It is easy to suggest that education of the patient is the answer, but not all patients are able to comprehend the choice, and in their desire to avoid pain they may push their practitioner into an approach that is against the patient's long-term interest. But if the practitioner understands the origin of a disease, he can give a clearer forecast, and may avoid the wrong treatment.

Causes of disease in traditional Chinese medicine may be summarized as follows:

1. Constitutional: pre-natal and hereditary factors, childhood and growth structure

xternal factors : weather and 'invisible worms'
nternal factors: emotions
4.   Abuse of qi
5.   Diet and drugs
6.   Wrong treatment.

1. Constitutional

Hereditary factors, as in Western medicines, can 'mark' our energy structure. In traditional Chinese medicine, still more important is the state of the parents' health at the conception of the child. Following that, the mother's health during pregnancy can be crucial. If she is poorly nourished, ill, or suffers from other problems such as trauma or over-use of drugs, the child will be affected, as it will also by a difficult delivery.

Astrologically it is hard to perceive racial or ancient hereditary factors, but aspects to Sun, Saturn and Moon, especially from Uranus, Neptune or Pluto, and the positions of these planets, may suggest qi potential at the time of conception. Until someone produces accurate conception birth data, we are still left with the birth chart! (Presumably, in the case of ova fertilized in a test-tube, other relevant factors will be the state of the parents' health at the time of donation of ovum or sperm.) The mother's contribution during pregnancy is best judged by consideration of Moon and Saturn, especially their mutual aspects. These planets respectively show the nourishment of the foetus and the structure being laid down, though it should be remembered that the genital code comes under Kidney, hence under Mercury, Sun, Neptune and Pluto, probably in that order.

Astrologers nowadays probe very deeply, seeking karmic causes if their clients are unwilling to accept more prosaic explanations. The chart encapsulates as far as it is able the energy at the moment of birth, crystallized as it were for that one moment. With Sun, Moon and eight planets, a paltry minimum of ten factors, the astrologer seeks to understand what the universe was thinking as it created the child. One is tempted to suggest that lacking more data, this is a quixotic gesture. Nevertheless, the fact remains that wherever a pattern is discernible, there is meaning for those who can grasp it. The larger the pattern, the further away one must be to discern it. Perhaps we are fortunate to possess just ten factors! In terms of gross malformation or disease in the new-born child, the chart is academic; the problems are all too apparent. For me, therefore, the chart is mainly useful in attempting to understand a patient's health during his life, not before it.

Early childhood is still dominated by Earth, Moon and Saturn; but Saturn's role, active perhaps during pregnancy, is more passive now; the body has been formed, and the four-phase cycle of life is now pulsing through it. Its nutrition is vital, however, and early aspects to the Moon and progressed Moon show how its needs are met. Unable to fend for itself, the child now looks outwards for security, and Saturn, formerly concerned with providing a mother in which to grow, and a structure to be grown, is now exteriorized into the family unit and its environment. Meanwhile, the growth pattern of learning how to be conscious, and then conscious learning, comes under Moon and increasingly Mercury, which via Kidney energy carries the inherited skills for life. If this vital early growth process is damaged, there may be left a profound imprint on the life. If the problem is one of lack of nourishment, then Moon and Saturn should reflect it. If growth is forced, intellectual attainments overemphasized, then Jupiter and Mercury will show it, as Wood will overstrain Water. As puberty approaches, overactive sexuality will strain Water, paving the way for early burn-out — another Mercury phenomenon.

If care is taken in childhood, with proper discipline and rest, good wholesome diet, a harmonious family and emotional life, then the pattern is set for later health on all levels. But insufficient rest strains Water (Mercury) and Earth (Saturn). Violence and anger disturb Wood (Jupiter), grief and loss strain Metal (Venus), and fever and too much hysterical laughing strain Fire (Mars). (To some extent, for women, there are two further periods after puberty when weakness can be turned — with proper care — into strength: pregnancy and menopause. Unfortunately the reverse is also true, and a woman who returns too quickly after delivery to active life may jeopardize her health for years. The same is true after miscarriage or abortion. Each of these periods marks an important new phase in the outflowing of the genetic code, and because of the importance of yin factors, notably Water and Earth, aspects to progressed Mercury, Moon and transiting Saturn will usually be prominent for strength or weakness.)

As we grow older, our spirit should manifest its solar inclinations more strongly. The Sun more than any other planet shows the point of our life, although it may focus its energy through another factor. But the extent to which it is able to manifest new life, to make changes for the better, is governed by the flexibility of the structure laid down by Moon, Mercury and Saturn. As we grow older, Saturn increasingly dominates and restricts as the Earth turns slowly leaden, heavy and tough. Illness then comes from inadaptability.

2. External factors
Having briefly considered the condition of the body, we can now look at some of the forces that impinge on it, always remembering that the stronger the inner energy, the more easily it will resist invasion, and the more violently it will confront any affront. Strong fevers suggest strong qi!

External factors are, with the main astrological significators, as follows. (The astrological significators will usually be transiting.)

(a) Wind   ♃, ☽, ♅.
(b) Cold   ♄, ☽, ☿.
(c) Heat and Fire   ♂, ☉.
(d) Damp   ♄, ♆, ☽, ♀.
(e) Dryness   ♂, ☿, ♃, ♅.

(a) *Wind* often spearheads disease, frequently combined with other factors. By *Wind* is meant not just the force of moving air, but sudden changes in weather. It includes draughts and air-conditioning. Its nature is moving: its effects migrate from one part of the body to another; a pain now here, now there. It comes on quickly, and being light and — apparently — insubstantial, it tends to show symptoms in the upper part of the body, head, shoulders, lungs, neck and the outer layers of the skin, through the pores of which it invades, to give, for example, the common cold. Like leaves in a wind, its nature is moving, so it gives tics, tremors, spasms and shakings. Typical symptoms are headaches, nasal obstruction, Bell's Palsy.

(b) *Cold* is the enemy of qi, so it reduces movement and heat. Its pain is aching, stabbing and localized, due to the fact that cold contracts muscles and stagnates movement, so that qi cannot move. What movement there is will be signs of cold: chills, shivering, sores. There may be numbness. Cold food is hard to digest and to warm, so symptoms of Spleen deficiency occur, e.g. undigested food in the stools.

(c) *Heat and Fire* occur in summer and under hot living or working conditions. To keep cool we need, like a refrigerator, a supply of cooling liquids and something to move them when they heat up. So extreme heat exhausts not only yin, but also qi. If yin is exhausted, yang becomes more powerful, so there is increased upward movement and dispersion. We go red in the face, sweat and get thirsty. There may be fever, restlessness, even delirium. Excess heat = *Fire* disturbs the blood and Liver by stirring up Wind, so Liver yang symptoms occur, and there may be skin rashes and haemorrhages, such as nose bleeds.

If untreated, other external factors can turn into *Fire*, as when we catch a cold which becomes a fever.

(d) *Damp* occurs in damp conditions, rainy seasons, and in damp surroundings e.g. living in a damp basement, sitting on damp grass, or working in a wet environment. Damp conditions are hard to shift: they feel, like a damp rag, very heavy. They make for tiredness and lassitude, as our qi tries to force movement through a damp fog of inertia. And, as in a damp fog, we feel heavy and confused; we have a blocked feeling in our heads, as if wrapped in a blanket. We may be dizzy and there is often anorexia, nausea and a feeling of fullness. Like a pocket of fog, damp tends to stick in a fixed place in the body, and many cases of rheumatism are due to it.

Damp is often chilly, but averse to too much heat. Where there is heat, there is usually a foul catarrh or discharge, yellow or green in colour: so we get leucorrhoea, abscesses, skin eruptions, fungal infections, nasal phlegm etc. The less heat there is, the more odourless and white are the discharges.

(e) *Dryness* dries out the fluids, initially of skin and lung. So the skin chaps easily, gets rough and cracks. Mouth, nose and throat lack moisture, and we may develop a yin-deficient cough: no sputum, irritating, with a sore throat. It occurs in dry desert-like areas, and in regions like central China, in late summer.

Invisible worms

The ancient Chinese managed to classify and treat diseases that we should describe as being due to bacteria and viruses. We in the West attack the disease by trying to kill the bug; the Chinese do so by altering its environment. But the ancient Chinese recognized that there were 'invisible worms', which caused what we would describe as epidemics. Although spread as it were by Wind, they affect large numbers of the population at the same time, so are less dependent on the individual's own environmental and life situation. In diagnosing these epidemics (such as measles, whooping cough, etc.) the symptoms are still usually classified as being due to Wind, and analysed into their constituent parts, e.g. Hot, Cold, Damp, Dry, Interior, Exterior, etc. The question is how prone is a particular individual to a particular type of disease, and this depends on his constitution. A hot type person with abundant yang is less likely to suffer from cold, and more likely to suffer from hot type diseases. Someone with a tendency to damp and warm type problems will be more likely to attract chickenpox (which likes those conditions) than his partner who is prone to cold damp conditions such as rheumatism.

In the case of deficiency type diseases, the method of treatment will be to warm and strengthen; in the case of excess type diseases, the method of treatment will be to attack the excess symptoms. But in nearly all cases the aim is to bring the organism back to health, on the assumption that a healthy body gives no succour to harmful invaders.

3. Internal factors
These are:

(a) Emotions.
(b) Internal Wind, Cold, Heat, Damp, Dryness, Fire.

(a) Emotions
These are a prominent cause of disease, especially in the West, where modern environmental control and nutrition to some extent reduce the danger from the external factors. Time and again, emotional imbalance seems to be the cause of a chronic and apparently — at least to Western medicine — incurable illness. One should not forget, however, that illness, from whatever cause, can also lead to an emotional imbalance, which may itself precipitate further illness.

(i) *Anger and frustration* are probably the most common causes of disease. They affect the Liver qi, leading to stuck Liver qi, Liver Fire, deficiency of Liver yin and Liver Blood, and a state in which Liver 'bullies' almost any other energy it can. As a rule it attacks Spleen/Stomach first, though this depends on the individual constitution. Astrological significators are ♃, ♅, ♂ and sometimes ☉.

Frustration tends to lead more to difficulties in other energies; anger more to effects on Liver Blood, Liver yin and Liver Fire. Frustration occurs when Saturn is strong or inhibiting, or Mars or Sun or Uranus weakly placed. Anger occurs when Jupiter combines with Mercury or Mars or is strongly placed, and Saturn or Moon less well placed. As one would expect from the four-phase diagram, a well-placed Venus counters the exaggerations and fulminations of a weak Jupiter, acting as it does across the cycle.

But anger that is long suppressed can reach out and attack Venus across the four-phase cycle, causing skin, respiratory and other chest problems.

Anger and frustration as causes need to be distinguished from irritability due to yin deficiency — especially Kidney yin deficiency. In this case we should expect to find strain on Mercury and perhaps Saturn.

(ii) *Joy, excitement, fright and shock* affect Fire, especially the Heart energy, so may if prolonged exhaust yin qi and Blood. They can produce a state of nervous hysteria and states bordering it, such as laughing and crying too frequently. Astrologically, this disturbance of the 'Shen' occurs in acute cases in accidents, when Mars and Uranus are prominent and challenging, and when Neptune and Venus are lulling us into a false sense of security. (For a fuller consideration of accidents, the reader is urged to read at least Carter's *The Astrology of Accidents*.) But wherever the shen is disturbed we should also expect some kind of Sun-Moon aspect.

In terms of symptoms, any Heart syndrome can appear. Where there has been prolonged worry, Spleen will also be weak, leading to formation of phlegm which 'obscures the orifices of the heart', hence mental disease, with manic behaviour, convulsions and delirium.

As effect, any prolonged weakening influence on yin or Blood may affect the Heart. Here look to the outer planets, notably Saturn, Neptune and Pluto in the case of overwork, whereas haemorrhage and fever come more under Mars and Sun.

See also under 'Fear' below.

(iii) *Overthinking and worry* affect Spleen qi and the Lungs. The qi 'coagulates' and then stagnates, leading to many deficient qi symptoms and Spleen/Stomach symptoms, such as tiredness, loss of appetite, poor digestion, desire for sweets and formation of phlegm.

Prominent astrologically are aspects of the Moon, Saturn and Venus.

(iv) *Grief and sadness* weaken Lung qi, hence all qi. If this grief can be expressed, the crying will open the lungs, generating qi; if it is suppressed, the lungs are compressed and insufficient air is breathed. If prolonged, it will damage Lung qi and Heart qi.

Saturn, Uranus, Moon and Neptune seem to occur most frequently.

If grief is suppressed for too long, then the reduction in qi may lead to stuck Liver qi. Indeed, one could say that the inability to express grief is a Liver symptom, as the Liver is responsible for the free expression of all emotion.

(v) *Fear* affects Heart and Kidney. Anticipatory anxiety, as before an exam, sends qi downwards to the area ruled by the Kidney, loosening its hold on the bladder and giving rise to sudden bowel movements.

Here the astrological association is with Sun, Mars and Mercury. In deeper states such as paranoia, the planet is Pluto or Saturn, whereas nameless fears come more under Neptune and Mercury. Sudden shocks can also be Jupiter-Uranus effects.

Anxiety about health comes also under Worry, so can involve Saturn or Mercury.

4. Abuse of qi

This includes overwork, fatigue, over- or under-exercise, excessive sex, and trauma.

The whole emphasis of Chinese medicine is on the correct understanding of qi. Although it is admitted that we possess physical bodies, even these are seen as merely more material or solidified forms of qi. Health consists in a free flow of adequate qi, which means suitable diet and hygiene, sufficient exercise and rest, proper breathing habits, forbearance and restraint in life's activities and opportunities, and the integration of spirit qi with physical qi, mind and body. We should learn to enjoy our *selves*.

Activities which impede this will injure qi and reduce health and life expectancy.

Overwork can be physical or mental. It may mean doing too many jobs at once, or overlong hours, overlifting, or just standing for too long and getting tired. The ensuing lack of qi leads to a lack of free flow of qi and signs of standstill: heaviness, aching, weakness, numbness and paralysis. This can occur locally or generally. Locally, for example, a young violinist in training had pain in the left arm and shoulder; a typist had neck problems; a housewife after spring-cleaning had general aching and a tennis elbow.

Exercise is necessary to keep qi circulating smoothly, but too much leads to exhaustion even if there are large muscles to show for it. Exhaustion should be balanced with adequate calm relaxation and sleep and massage to move qi through the exhausted tissues. Under-exercise is harmful too; zangfu lose their ability to maintain free flow of qi, giving poor resistance to disease and lack of self-confidence.

Too much sex drains Kidney jing, sex here being understood to be sperm - hence the Chinese practice of ejaculatory restraint. But it can also drain a woman whose ecstatic spasms in excess drain Kidney qi and eventually jing. (For symptoms of deficient Kidney jing and qi see Chapter 5.) For many women, giving birth to and bringing up a large family may also drain jing. Like all healthy activities, the union of male with female can also strengthen qi and integrate personality, but not when indulged in to excess.

Trauma is similar to overwork in some ways, in that it drains qi and leads to stagnation, as any bruise will testify. The more qi there is initially, the less the effect. The less qi, as in ill, old or weakened patients, the greater the effect, because they have less power to repair the damage. The trauma can also affect the Heart, because of the shock and fright.

Astrologically there are two sides to this question. In the body there are many kinds of qi that may be affected.

First, Mercury represents Kidney qi, although the Sun, Pluto and Neptune are aspects of it. This is the source of energy that we use to keep us going when we are exhausted. It is the energy represented by our genetic code, our last ditch. When it is used up, we die. This source is drained by overwork with lack of calm rest, over-fatigue, too much sex, or too big a family, and where there is shock, or where in spite of injury we force ourselves to continue.

Secondly, Moon and Saturn (Earth) are different levels of our strength, derived from adequate nutrition and exercise. Saturn concerns the physical body, Moon its good working order. Sun and, to a lesser extent, Mars (Fire) denote our spirit and fortitude, the shen that is shaken or dislodged by, for example, trauma. The quality of our musculature is partly represented by Venus (Metal) which also denotes the value we place upon it (as it represents the value we place upon so many other factors). Moon and Venus and Mercury represent our intestines, through which we absorb food. Moon is their general working order, Venus (Metal) their power to eliminate and to absorb, whereas Mercury (Water) is mainly how they respond when we are challenged. (There is a relationship here to how well we know ourselves.) Jupiter (Wood) shows our ability to recover. Uranus is our ability to change dramatically, usually by choice or conscious understanding of the process. Neptune can represent our ability to absorb qi abuse without apparently showing it. (What actually happens is that we absorb it on a different level which, although less obvious, takes longer to work out. This level is often that of Heart and Kidney.)

The astrological indicators of abuse of qi work usually by transit, the main exception being progressions of Sun and Moon which bring to the surface the complex psychological patterns indicated by natal positions. These natal complexes show any tendency to overwork, to taking several jobs at once, insecurity or greed (for example), and a progression or transit sparks it off. Progressed Moon brings to the surface problems associated with the past, our automatic and unconscious inclinations; progressed Sun points to situations which we have more control over, though the sacrifices may be great.

Transiting Jupiter gives new openings, new friends and for many people, frustration, anger and the need to compromise, especially if expectation exceeds reality. It can mean doing two jobs at once, or moving house, marrying or divorcing. We are being asked to move on, and as we usually cling to the past, we try to do too much, and exhaust ourselves.

Transits of Uranus act rather like Jupiter, but there is more shock to them, with consequent sudden demands on Kidney. If there is a sexual element in the transit, there may be strain on Kidney jing! But Uranus allows us to project our personality in a new way, so we often rise to the challenge, which excites and fascinates us. On the other hand, we may just have too much to do. Jupiter and Uranus encourage us to experiment and to eat too much. If we get tired and overeat, we end up with a cold. (Transits of Uranus usually give the author a cold!)

Mars transits help us to express ourselves freely, for the joy of it. They may therefore lead to opposition or, in those who have been led to believe that no weakness is admissible, they can lead to crude, overbearing, daring or heedless behaviour.

Saturn transits can be great opportunities for growth: it is the body and all its needs which are ready to move on. Unfortunately, Saturn also brings the probability of reduction of existing standards of life. The harder we cling to them, the harder we must work. So Saturnian transits are often dreaded because they seem to limit us. Physically they show our limitations.

Venus and Mercury transits are probably effective in their own way, but I have not found them particularly useful. Much the same applies to Sun transits.

Neptune transits lead to dissipation of energy from one level to another. Neptune seems to abort progress or push it in an unwanted direction. Usually there is a subtly fatiguing anxiety which strains Kidney qi. The influence of drugs and alcohol, and of Neptune, is to falsify a situation, to suppress the symptoms. A (Neptune) drug is mainly used as a means of dispersing yang and of strengthening yin, but when the drug is discontinued, the emotional life is at best no better than when the drug was begun, and the patient is left in addition with the problems of withdrawal and addiction. Neptune drugs do not seem to tonify or strengthen; they do, however, suppress symptoms, eventually reducing the body's ability to mend itself. (This applies mainly to long-term treatment; few people would forgo the benefit of a Neptunian anaesthetic during an operation.) The other problem with Neptune is that its transits drain all three leg-yin zang organs, Spleen, Kidney and Liver, though its effect is more noticeable when transiting Saturn (Spleen), Mercury (Kidney) and Jupiter (Liver). Thus in transits of Saturn it seems to weaken the quality of the physical body, digestion and qi: transiting Mercury, we get genito-urinal complaints and fears of impotence or infertility. Transiting Venus it brings sadness and grief, influenza and bronchial complaints, and an accumulation of phlegm.

Transits by Pluto are more strengthening, if we can survive them! They take a long time, so it is less easy to be sure of their effect, but they seem to bring to the surface new characteristics from our genetic code, forcing out the outworn, in whichever zangfu is represented by the planet transited.

5. Diet and drugs

Spleen and Stomach produce qi and Blood from our diet. We can abuse this source by overeating, undereating, eating food that is too cold and chills Spleen yang, eating food that is too hot, spicy, rich or alcoholic and produces phlegm and heat, or by eating unclean food or food with too little variety. Eating when neither calm nor relaxed also impedes digestion, as does eating while working or reading. Returning to work too soon after eating can reduce absorption and lead to congestion.

In traditional Chinese medicine the tastes which are associated with the zangfu are as follows:

♃	Liver	Sour	
♂	Heart	Bitter	A desire for the
♄	Spleen	Sweet	associated taste often
♀	Lung	Pungent	occurs when the zangfu
☿	Kidney	Salty	is out of balance.

Yin	Salty, bitter, sour:	Makes energy go down, e.g. bitter taste is often diuretic, sour taste quells anger.
Yang	Sweet, pungent:	moves energy upwards. e.g. curry energizes and produces heat; sweet food warms and nourishes.

Disease caused by poor diet or drugs is hard to cure with acupuncture until the diet is altered or the drug discontinued. Drugs here include abuse of drugs, and vaccination, often a source of disease.

10.

ASSOCIATIONS WITH THE ZODIAC

For many, this chapter will seem the easiest. It is, however, the least useful in diagnosing disease, and should be looked upon as mainly speculative.

The fact that there are twelve meridians and twelve signs of the Zodiac has led astrologers to seek equivalents. Here is the usual scheme:

TABLE 1.

Sign Ruler	Meridians	Phase	Time
♈ Aries ♂	Lung	} Metal	3-5 a.m.
♉ Taurus ♀	Large Intestine		5-7 a.m.
♊ Gemini ☿	Stomach	} Earth	7-9 a.m.
♋ Cancer ☽	Spleen		9-11 a.m.
♌ Leo ☉	Heart	} Fire	11 a.m.-1 p.m.
♍ Virgo ☿	Small Intestine		1-3 p.m.
♎ Libra ♀	Bladder	} Water (Yin)	3-5 p.m.
♏ Scorpio ♂, ♇	Kidney		5-7 p.m.
♐ Sagittarius ♃	Pericardium	} Water (Yang)	7-9 p.m.
♑ Capricorn ♄	Three Heater	or Fire	9-11 p.m.
♒ Aquarius ♄, ♅	Gall Bladder	} Wood	11 p.m.-1 a.m.
♓ Pisces ♃, ♆	Liver		1-3 a.m.

This has the happy advantage that the meridians follow each other in the order in which qi proceeds along them, commencing at Lung Meridian.

There are a number of suggestive connections. Taurus is ruled by Venus, which rules Metal phase; Cancer is ruled by the Moon, associated with the Earth phase; Leo is ruled by the Sun, associated partly with Fire phase; Scorpio is ruled by Pluto, associated partly with Water phase; Pisces is ruled by Jupiter, which rules Wood phase.

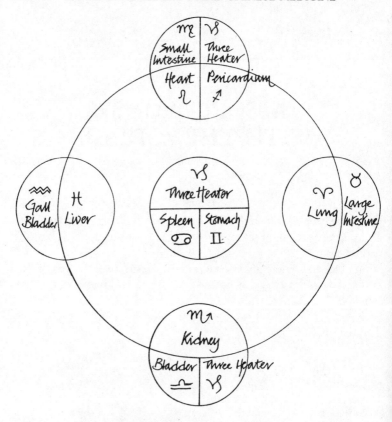

Diagram 6. The twelve meridians.

Diagram 6 shows one way of arranging the twelve meridians; it places Three-Heater on its three levels, upper, middle and lower chou. (Roughly these are chest, epigastrium and upper abdomen, lower abdomen.)

Another, more common scheme is shown in Diagram 7.

In the 'sheng' diagram (on page 161), energy flows clockwise in normal health. Thus the Fire phase transmits power to Earth, then to Metal and so on. The most useful insight here is the rulership by Mercury of Water phase, Gemini (Stomach) and Virgo (Small Intestine). Equating a Mercurial imbalance with a state of anxiety, and a desire to acquire information to assuage that anxiety, we see how appetite increases (Stomach) for both news and food when Water (Mercury) is deficient. When anxiety becomes tension and approaches panic, we get intestinal butterflies, sudden urges to defecate and urinate,

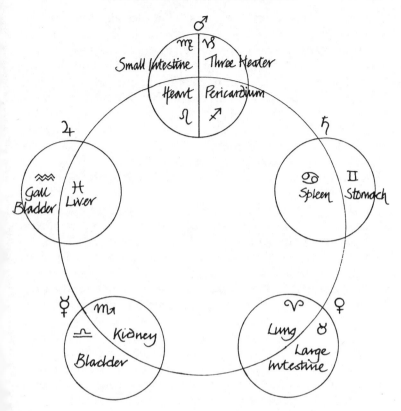

Diagram 7. Sheng cycle.

increased or decreased thirst or hunger — all symptoms of an upset Earth phase. If we lose control of ourselves, our powers of discrimination (Small Intestine) go, affecting the Heart through the relationship between Heart (Leo) and Small Intestine (Virgo), coupled energies in the Fire phase. The poor digestions of many nervous or self-critical or worrying people are another facet, as is the inability of many such to put on good healthy muscle tissue. There is a message here! Mercury and Moon rule Gemini (Stomach) and Cancer (Spleen) in Earth phase, the phase that gives a reliable body. If we cannot relax, and worry too much (over-thinking weakens the Spleen/Stomach), our bodies cannot grow healthy, and we shall need to draw on deeper energies (Water phase). Here then is another approach to the idea that digestion is affected by the mind.

Exploring the diagram further, Metal receives its energy from Earth.

If we have an upset digestion, we shall not feel comfortable with
ourselves, we may suffer from constipation or its opposite, our skins
suffer and, particularly if we have eaten too much rich food, we may
get catarrh, which lodges in our nose, throat and possibly lungs as
'cold'. Here Metal energy, which is our first defence against external
influences, is weakened. What is more, we begin to smell foul to others,
if not to ourselves. We become no longer a beautiful, valuable object
(Metal-Venus). At the same time, anyone with acute constipation
and a cold up his nose (i.e. Metal problems), is going to find it more
difficult to assert himself, though he may well be more selfish (Aries).
How can you speak firmly and clearly with a sore throat and phlegm
in your bronchi?

And how in that condition can you rest (Water)! Unless Large
Intestine can absorb water from the faeces at the correct rate, we
shall have either too much or too little urine, so our blood will be
either too rich or too dilute and we shall be either toxic or oedematous
(*pace* those with a knowledge of physiology!). Venus rules Taurus
(Large Intestine) and Libra (Bladder) and the interconnection between
Metal and Water phase continues with Mars' rulership of both Aries
(Lung) and Scorpio (Kidney). Lung energy is said to 'regulate the
water passages', both in terms of sweat and of superfluous body fluid
sent to the Kidney. But there is another, and interesting, relationship.
Water phase imbalance can show symptoms of fear, anxiety, tension
and boredom (another form of tension); Metal energy (via Aries —
Lung) is the *only* phase over which we can all exert conscious control
without need of biofeedback or yogic training, by regulating our
breathing. In this regulation of breathing we have a means of
controlling those Water symptoms. (Every smoker knows this: watch
the delicate increase of tension as the cigarette is prepared, then lit.
Finally, with the first smooth inspiration and sighing - occasionally
'shuddering'! - exhalation, the energy is sent down to Kidney. Release
of tension, smile on lips. The advertisements would have you believe
that it is the tobacco! Forget it. Tobacco makes you sick and is an
addictive poison; learn to breathe properly and you will control your
tension!)

Note also, that if our breathing is calm and relaxed, we shall be
so too: so our digestion (Earth — mother energy of Metal) will be
strengthened.

Aries (Lung) and Libra (Bladder) are opposite signs, so are Taurus
(Large Intestine) and Scorpio (Kidney). Wood and Water phases are
connected through their associated signs, by trine, hence element
— Air for Bladder and Gall Bladder; Water element for Kidney and

Liver. Hence these phases should work closely together as they have much in common. Drugs, for example, affect them both; many Liver syndromes affect or may be caused by weak Water. If we wake in the night — often a Water problem — the Liver cannot properly store Blood and we awaken in the morning unrefreshed. Bladder and Gall Bladder meridians control Back and Sides of the body, the yang areas, and a problem along one meridian can often be alleviated by treating the other. On another level, perhaps one could say that the power and self-discipline that goes with a strong Scorpio individual is a necessary pre-requisite if one is to be free to experience life safely as a Piscean explorer. One must be centred.

The same is true for Wood and Fire phases, but a true Leo (Heart) needs to be able to appreciate the feelings of the people. He needs Pisces behind him for support. And Pisceans and Leonians are both traditionally associated with acting, surely one of the most yang professions! The reader is invited to consider further relationships in the sheng cycle.

Next we will consider, briefly, the ke or ko cycle, illustrated by Diagram 8.

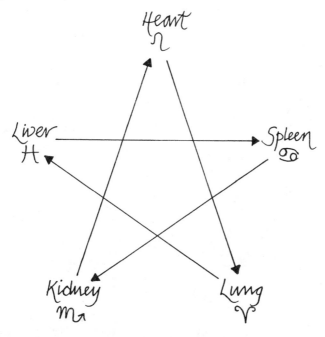

Diagram 8. 'Ke' diagram.

The ke cycle is one of control. Water phase controls Fire; Metal controls Wood. In reverse, we get the wu cycle, where Fire insults Water, Wood insults Metal, etc. (In acupuncture this controlling cycle is often most important, although I believe that more insight is gained from the four-phase diagram as to both control, balance and insult.)

How we use the cycle in daily life is exemplified by the Metal-Wood control. If we are angry, we shall assert ourselves more effectively if our breathing is rhythmic and controlled. Here Metal controls Wood. Equally, if we are shy, then steady, deep breathing will calm our nerves (Water) and control the way we project ourselves (Wood). The interesting thing about these two is that Liver passes its energy to Lung along the meridian pathway. So Liver both feeds, and is controlled by, Lung. Many cases of deficient qi (Lung) come from frustration (Liver), and opening the acupuncture meridian points connecting these meridians can, in the right circumstances, be profoundly effective.

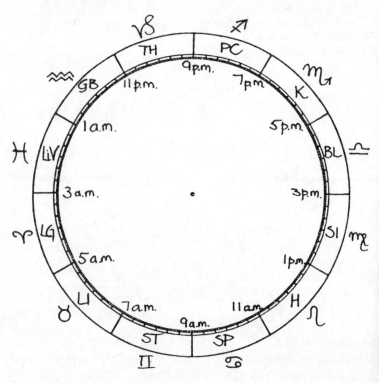

Diagram 9.   Meridian times and Natural Houses.

Although Diagram 9 is not how traditional Chinese medicine views time, astrologers may find it easier than Diagram 10. I have certainly found that emphasis in a chart on a particular house, as opposed to sign, can occasionally point to problems with the associated zangfu organ or meridian, but this is not a fixed rule. Nearly always it is a planet that, by position or aspect, gives a better indication. Planets in the house opposite can also be pointers. For example, Carter noted that heart attacks had occurred in charts where the ruler of the 5th house was in the 11th. Scrutiny of Diagram 7 indicates a relationship between Gall Bladder and Heart where Gall Bladder on the outer sheng cycle nourishes Small Intestine: if it fails, problems can arise with Small Intestine's paired organ, Heart. Readers will note similar situations elsewhere in Diagram 7, which seems to indicate that because of the clockwise flow there is some likelihood of problems occurring on this basis in the following situations.

Ruler of 7th house lies in 1st.
Ruler of 8th house lies in 2nd.
Ruler of 3rd house lies in 9th.
Ruler of 4th house lies in 10th.
Ruler of 5th house lies in 11th.
Ruler of 6th house lies in 12th.

The reverse is less true.

It is tempting to draw similar conclusions from Diagram 8 (ke cycles) and the reader may wish to examine charts where the ruler of, say, the 5th house (Heart) lies in the 8th, and vice versa.

Signs are a problem, and are less reliable indicators of associated organ or meridian weakness, although the Ascendant, Sun and Moon signs are often useful. I have found they point more to a particular phase energy (e.g. Fire, Earth) that may show weakness according to the sheng, ke or wu cycle. Thus someone with an emphasis in Cancer in the 1st house may suffer from Earth phase problems where the main causative factor is deficiency of qi due to overwork, such qi deficiency being consonant with Metal — Lung deficiency, indicating a background of grief, disappointment or loss, driving the native (from Aries house — Lung) to compensate, but unable to exert sufficient control over Wood via the ke cycle. Wood, therefore, becomes overactive and invades Earth, causing duodenal ulcers. It is in this way that the sheng cycle can be revealing when used with signs or, better, houses.

In the hope that too much information will not be unnecessarily

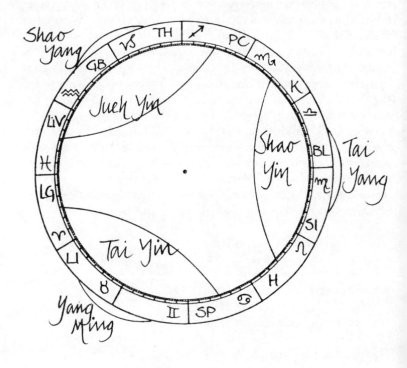

Diagram 10.   The Six Divisions.

confusing, there are other important connections between the meridians, one of which is called 'the Six Divisions', shown in Diagram 10. The use of the Six Divisions is beyond the scope of this book, dealing with, amongst other matters, the progress of a disease from one level inwards or outwards. It is relevant here, however, because it gives a different form of pairing, indicating a closer relationship between the ways certain energies work than might otherwise be apparent. Thus Small Intestine and Bladder are closely related in terms of their meridian flow, and because problems in one easily cause problems in the other. Notice that Heart and Kidney, although not directly related by meridian flow on the surface, are connected by a deep meridian; more important (as the four-phase diagram shows by polarity), there is a close interconnection in the way they function, which Western medicine has not been slow to realize.

Although Three Heater has no clearly defined organ, its meridian and that of Gall Bladder are frequently useful in treating problems on the side of the body. There are also a number of acupuncture points on the Three Heater meridian that are useful for treating Gall Bladder and Liver problems, for example pain in the side, on the flanks or intercostal, and intestinal congestion. Sagittarius is usually associated with liver and thigh problems (to name but a few!) Diagram 10 gives more credibility to this, as Pericardium (Sagittarius) and Liver (Pisces) are closely related, and although the Pericardium meridian flows only down to the bowels (on its inner level), the Liver and Gall Bladder meridians flow over the thigh. In cases of sciatica and lumbo-sacral pain, meridians often effective are Gall Bladder, Bladder, Pericardium and Three Heater.

However, as mentioned before, it is the planets ruling the signs that are important. Readers may care to tabulate the sign rulers of

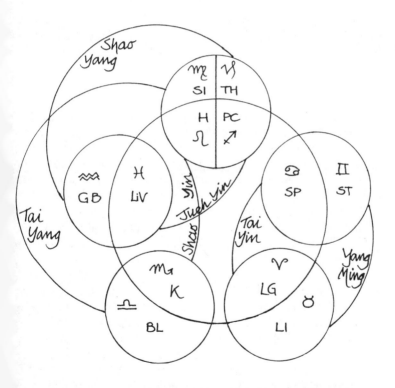

Diagram 11. The Six Divisions.

the six divisions with a view to examining the relevant planets in their charts.

Placing these divisions on the sheng diagram we get Diagram 11.

Although Water-Fire, Wood-Fire and Earth-Metal are closely related, there is no connection between, say, Fire-Metal or Metal-Water. To some extent one may account for this by saying that Earth and Metal are so important on their own account that they need no help! There are other meridians that come between them (eight extra meridians), but these are beyond the scope of this work.

Twenty-Four Hour Clock

Energy in the meridians flows from one to the next at the indicated time. At its horary time (e.g. Heart 11 a.m.-1 p.m.) the related zangfu organ is said to be particularly energized and susceptible to treatment, unlike its opposite time (11 p.m.-1 a.m. = Gall Bladder) when the organ's energy is dormant. Readers with health problems that occur always at a particular hour of the day may find these times illuminating, but they should always consider in addition the zangfu organ whose time is opposite. Thus problems at 11 p.m.-1 a.m. may be Liver; they could also be Heart.

Astrologers have a problem: they count the houses from times that on average approximate to 6 a.m., noon, 6 p.m. and midnight. Traditional Chinese medicine counts the two-hour periods from the 'odd' hours. This may lend credibility to the theory that the house cusps are in fact points of maximum effect, and that each house begins some time before its cusp. Traditional Chinese medicine practitioners frequently note problems that begin at about the time expected of the relevant zangfu, however. For instance, Water phase problems not infrequently occur between 3 p.m. and 7 p.m., peaking at 5 p.m.

Clinically the law of midday-midnight is often most useful. From an astrological point of view, it proceeds in the opposite direction to the houses, following the apparent movement of the sun and planets round the Earth. It is useful when particular chart emphasis lies over the organ horary time. Thus, emphasis in the 10th house when linked with other factors can lead to the symptoms of Heart problems such as palpitations, flushing, panicky feelings and tremor. But such problems are usually Heart-Kidney, not just Heart, so one would expect to find, for example, prominent aspects from $\yen$ or P. Such aspects, I have found, are by no means always the challenging ones. (In one case, for example, there was $\odot_{10} \, \sigma \, \yen_{10} \, \star \, P_{12}$ with $\mathcal{D}$ alone by quadrant in the 5th house, and $\odot/\mathcal{D} = P$. As all

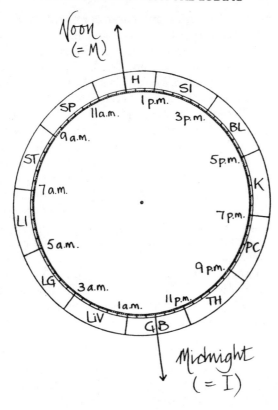

Diagram 12. 24 Hour Clock.
Law of Midday-Midnight.

astrologers know, there are usually a mass of indicators for a particular syndrome if one is prepared to look for them, and able to see them.) But as always, this way of using the information is less useful than direct consideration of the planets themselves. The angles, planets, Sun and Moon are the important factors; signs and houses are less significant.

Diagram 12 gives an alternative view of the houses. The 1st and 2nd houses, being Metal, govern our skin and appearance, the first impact we make on our environment. If we value ourselves, we have a positive approach. A difficult persona conceals all sorts of problems. (Homoeopaths will note that Psora, the original miasm that arose from suppression, is classically related to an itch on the *skin*.) At birth we must breathe qi to live. Next we need nourishment (10th and 11th houses), later in life we seek support from our friends and colleagues, in association with those around us from whom we have to make a living. By this stage our personalities are developing and we need attention; we have to learn to shine (Medium Coeli: 9th and 10th houses), then to learn and digest (8th and 9th) and discriminate and teach. The 8th house (Bladder) gives reserves and flexibility (Water phase), but is in the 6th and 7th (Kidney) that we are to balance ourselves with those around us. Through this house we connect racially (inherited genes) with those around us; without colleagues we cannot continue the human race. Their opposition may evoke fear or anxiety in us (Water phase), and compensating qualities, antagonism, desire for power, both highly Scorpionic. Whereas we eliminate in our faeces the food that we cannot absorb (Large Intestine, 1st house), in the 7th house via Kidney we eliminate the fluids within us that we have manufactured and now return, enriched. What we give and receive on the Kidney level is deeper and less capable of conscious control. By choosing what we eat, we exert some conscious control over our faeces. It takes a much deeper awareness, derived usually from long experience of mankind, of our world and our Maker for us to purify ourselves (Kidney — 7th house). When we are clear, clean, pure, we leave no mark on the world, save that of pure emptiness.

The nature of Pericardium is traditionally that of Ambassador for the Heart (see the 'The Officials', page 171), so this paradigm makes the 5th house the area of joyous expression of ourselves, the fun, laughter and wisdom we bring to our relationships. The Pericardium relates to the area round the Heart and, in traditional Chinese medicine, to the diaphragm, free movement of which is needed in laughing and breathing deeply. The more deeply we breathe, the more profoundly we move our diaphragm, and the more we take energy down to the hara, the lower abdominal area which is the centre of our reserves, governed by Kidney.

The Three Heater can be coupled with Pericardium; also via Shao yang, with Gall Bladder and Liver. In its relationship with Pericardium, it suggests that all these 'burning' spaces are involved when we breathe and laugh healthily and deeply, that individuals with much chart emphasis in that area (4th and 5th houses) should be particularly careful to maintain good habits, the free flow of energy through all parts of their systems.

The houses covered by Three Heater, Gall Bladder and Liver are the period around midnight, when overactivity (Wood) can ruin restful sleep. The Chinese have a high opinion of some of the first

English they met; they said that they had good 'Gall', meaning courage, nerve and, by implication, decisiveness — qualities derived perhaps from a hardy upbringing in a challenging but safe environment where the emphasis was on the foundations of rectitude, King or Queen and country, with an adventurous spirit: individuals who believed they were 'Right'!

The Liver's houses (2nd and 3rd) make it the area for exploring and expanding consciousness through learning and movement. Too much going on in the mind inhibits sleep at these times.

The above is but a brief introduction!

The Officials

Chinese medicine is very pragmatic: if one paradigm of the pathology of an illness doesn't work, try another. This explains why this chapter contains a number of different methods.

One such paradigm is the idea of the 'Officials'. Each of the orbs of energy is given a different personality, describing its function. Imagine in ancient China, an Emperor. He may not be seen, but he is there! He exerts his authority through his officials, first of whom is the Sovereign Prince (Heart-Sun-Leo), who maintains individuality and is ultimately responsible for keeping the nation, or the person, integrated. Assisting the Prince is a Prime Minister (Lungs-Mars-Aries) on whom rhythmic order depends. This would be the day-to-day running of the kingdom, from supply to demand, from start to finish, keeping wheels oiled, with initiative to send energy wherever needed, ensuring that everything goes along quietly and in order, that the pulse of life flows smoothly. He is rather like a central government that regulates activities throughout the kingdom by upholding a reliable legal pattern for all.

The Prince has a strategic planner and general in charge of armed forces (Liver-Jupiter-Pisces) who has the job of maintaining a cheerful optimistic disposition in the country. Through continual planning and revision he accrues, renews and assembles forces, according to the needs of rest or action, acting as troubleshooter. His job of keeping the people cheerful and defending the kingdom brings him into close contact with the Ambassador (Pericardium-Jupiter-Sagittarius), who protects the Prince from tiresome outside pressures.

The Minister of Domestic Affairs and Trade Unions (Spleen-Moon-Cancer) has an important function, acting through the people as a calming central influence. He is closer to the people than any other Minister save the Prince. He overlooks food and transport systems, water supplies and the communications network. He calms the others and enables them to act, although he is their servant. In constant touch with all parts of the system, he is the earth on which they all stand and from which each receives his energy and nourishment. It is for his good that they work.

Last of the six main Ministers is the Minister of Rest and Play (Kidney-Mars/Pluto-Scorpio) whose job is harder to understand. Without him there would be no reason for life, and no way of continuing the species. As he carries the blueprints of the nation, he is also minister of genealogy, history and heraldry. He stores knowledge of handicrafts, technical skills and education, and he knows how to concentrate force to achieve a desired aim. He represents the will of the people to persevere. (Not to be confused with 'the Will of the People', a concept from another paradigm!) All the roots of the organism originate with him. He is like a foundation stone, but also a place of retreat, where individuals go to collect and concentrate their energies.

Each Minister has an assistant, who may at times seem more important or more energetic, and who frequently covers more ground.

Minister	Assistant	Assistant's Job
Prince (Heart)	Small Intestine (☿ — Virgo)	To receive, assimilate and separate pure from impure. The Prince's secretariat. (Spy network?)
Prime Minister (Lung)	Large Intestine (♀ — Taurus)	Temporary storage and disposal of rubbish. (Publicity Officer?)
Strategic Planner (Liver)	Gall Bladder (♄ — Aquarius)	Decision and direction. (Commander of offensive forces?)
Domestic Affairs (Spleen)	Stomach (☿ — Gemini)	Intermediate storage, Imports. Energy distribution and nourishment.
Rest and Play (Kidney)	Bladder (♀ — Libra)	General assembly. Controls reserves. Very wide power of supply. Exports.
Ambassador (Pericardium)	Three Heater (♄ — Capricorn)	Good communications. A source of constructive energy.

No analogy is perfect — certainly not this one! Some functions are shared between officials; some officials seem to get their fingers into everything. But this is simply one view of the body's energy, useful at times. A particular official pressure can show symptoms correlating with the nature of his duties. So if Gall Bladder is in disarray, we may be unable to take effective decisions, and we may be over — or under-aggressive.

The idea of a kingdom may not suit you, in which case picture instead a sailing vessel, its Captain (Heart), First Mate (Lung), Planning Officer (Liver), Personnel and Supplies Officer (Spleen), Cargo Officer (Kidney) — more active in port than at sea, where he has to entertain the passengers — Communications Officer (Pericardium), Captain's Sidekick (Small Intestine), Navigator (Gall Bladder), Cook and Librarian (Stomach), Storeman (Bladder) and Engineer and Handyman (Three Heater).

The passenger owns the vessel, built it, and is trying to become a better human being, so he doesn't have much time for chores, and apart from Captain and Cargo Officer, nobody sees much of him. The remaining individual — Rubbish Disposal, Water Purification and Painter (Large Intestine) — is sometimes not spoken to by the others as much as he should be, because he tends to smell a bit. But he is an interesting fellow, easy to relate to, who saves what he earns and has invested some of it in the vessel and its cargo, so he cannot be ignored. He is a strong man in a fight and looks splendid in uniform. He is thinking of joining Friends of the Earth. He runs the ship's shop and acts as Purser. First Mate (Lung) and Purser (Large Intestine), look after the sailing gear and rigging.

This gives a flavour to the twelve meridians; they each now have a personality. Astrologically, if a planet is in, say, high focus, consider which meridian and personality it symbolizes. Counselling the native on the needs and obligations of that personified meridian is sometimes highly conducive to greater self-awareness.

11.

CONCLUDING NOTES

Chinese medicine is a vast subject, at least in its ramifications. But in principle it is simple, compared with its Western counterpart. It uses concepts that are basic and readily grasped by an uncomplicated mind, because they fit human experience. A long tradition, its roots in folk medicine, has been accompanied by a growing philosophical, not to say metaphysical, awareness. Over several thousand years, this produced minds that were at their peak, intellectual, pragmatic, intuitive, sensible to their feelings.

More than we can easily appreciate in the West, there is a strong feeling for life as it once was in the 'Golden Era', the olden times of the ancestors. Even the insistent demands of communism have hardly obliterated a deep reverence for the ancestral gods, whether they be one's forefathers, or wrapped up in the ineffable essence of Tao. Where they can, Chinese the world over practise daily the meditative movements of Qigong and Tai Qi. With their quiet, deft, unhurried movements they centre themselves within the Tao. They move with a fluid grace, representing the animals of their mythology, the anger and hopes of their heroes. Then they are ready for daily life, steady in their energy, minds alert and uncluttered.

The history of traditional Chinese medicine has had, like that of China, many vicissitudes. Think of the civilizing effect of its vast systems of irrigation, and of what happens to these systems when threatened by outside forces, whether meteorological, political or epidemic. Any one part affects in some measure every other part, just as natural springs lose their force when tapped elsewhere, or as a blocked gutter pipe can have consequences out of all proportion to the cause. To forestall disaster needs planning. Too long spent planning leaves no time to achieve one's aims; too little, and manual effort is wasted.

The development of the ability to plan ahead, to administer

effectively, must have occurred relatively early at a time when, from the desperate needs of survival predating civilization, there remained a strong awareness of the learned roles that differentiated the functions of 'male' and 'female', let us say. One became more concerned with children, agriculture and the continuation of the species through care and nourishment; the other became more responsible for food gathering by hunting, defence and appropriation. *His* life was more likely to be spent in exploration of the outer universe, *hers* in the inner one. Whereas she had to conform and maintain the status quo, he could break away and grow as an individual. His activities were more on the outside — they required force and vigour, warmth, noise and movement; hers concerned the inside — control, steadiness, nourishment, reserves, a place to rest, to recuperate, to be healed, to grow in peace. Such specialization leads to faster development, but it also brings conflict as each tries to assert its importance. In these conditions there grew the Chinese preoccupation with balance, mythologized in the 'Golden Era', and the desire to rebalance, epitomized by the vast irrigation system.

A modern view might be that primitive awareness is more right brain hemisphere centred, being pattern-orientated, intuitive and imaginative (so also more paranoid, religiously suspicious and cruel), whereas the logical planning functions are more left brain hemisphere centred (so can be blind to the wider, non-material implications, and more ruthless) and that there existed in China a time when they flourished together. Only such a combination might have the insight to perceive the irrigatory channels of life in the body, and the consciousness to explore and map them.

As part of their observation of the universal tides, the Chinese developed their astrology as one way of understanding the flux of life. It has some similarities to its Western counterpart, and relies heavily on cycles, especially of Sun and Moon. They observed the planets and correlated them with certain phases of experience, but from there the tracks diverged: the Chinese symbol combinations differing markedly in method, thought and spirit from Western astrology, which became more mathematically precise. The spirit of Chinese astrology resides in an understanding of myths, just as in the West. The Chinese language is ideographic, more right-brained, than Western writing, and they think more by superimposing images, whereas we think more by describing things in detail. We therefore know all about something, but lose its flavour. It is hard for us to understand their continual blurring of images unless we grow more right brain hemisphere strength. The reason for this book is that, because the Chinese astrological mythology is less accessible to us, and because we have developed in Western astrology our own mythology and right-brained methods, it is more useful for us to compare our own astrology with the Chinese medical model of life than to attempt first to understand their astrology, useful though that may be.

The basic awareness of being human is not so different, West and East. But the Chinese description of illness gives its flavour much more clearly and can be grasped more easily than the Western medical model. They speak of 'cold', 'damp', 'heat', and these are common in experience. What a pity that Western medicine has lost contact with these vital observations. Too often, patients suffer from Western prescribed drugs or foods because the doctor failed to realize that the illness was, say, of a 'cold' type, and he prescribed a drug which 'cooled'. Better surely to give a drug that 'warms'! Only a few centuries ago, all apothecaries were conversant with these descriptions of disease, as also with Western astrology, and we have a venerable tradition of herbal medicine which has explored these images, as anyone who has read Culpeper will be aware. (It may be added that if Western herbalism loses contact with these common observations of life in an attempt to become more scientifically acceptable, it will go the same way as Western medicine, losing its soul and its humanity.)

However, astrologers have a great advantage: they are used to associating, to seeing order through a blur of different energies. The system introduced here requires the learning of only a few more sets of associations (at least initially), all common in life, and not difficult to grasp even — it is hoped — by non-astrologers. Those energies are related to the planets and this book is an introduction to that relationship.

Our astrology is a home-grown right brain hemisphere product, useful in many spheres, from psychology to politics. However, because of the way Western medicine has chosen to go, Western astrology has lost contact with some of the commonest experiences of life, of energy and of illness. We speak of astrology as being capable of describing the whole; it should therefore be possible to relate illness to personality, and the Chinese model can be our guide. In the final analysis, we can throw away our ephemeris, as the Chinaman throws out his I Ching, and see what needs to be done directly. Until then, let us enjoy the riches our astrology can contribute to the game.

APPENDIX

5 Phase Associations

	JUPITER	MARS	SATURN	VENUS	MERCURY
Planet	JUPITER	MARS	SATURN	VENUS	MERCURY
Phase	WOOD	FIRE	EARTH	METAL	WATER
Direction	East	South	Centre	West	North
Season	Spring	Summer	(late summer)	Autumn	Winter
Climate	Windy	Hot	Damp	Dry	Cold
Emotion	Anger	Joy	Over-thinking	Grief	Fear
Sound	Shouting	Laughing	Singing	Weeping	Groaning
Orifice	Eyes	Tongue	Mouth	Nose	Ears
Yin organ	Liver	Heart	Spleen	Lungs	Kidney
Yang organ	Gall Bladder	Small Intestine	Stomach	Large Intestine	Bladder
Tissue	Tendons	Blood Vessels	Flesh	Skin and Body Hair	Bones
Smell	Rancid	Burnt	Fragrant	Rank	Putrid
Taste	Sour	Bitter	Sweet	Pungent	Salty
Colour	Green	Red	Yellow	White	Blue-black
Power	Give Birth	Mature assertion	Calmly neutralize	Refine, make Space	Sustain
Time	11p.m.-3a.m.	11a.m.-3p.m. 7p.m.-11p.m.	7a.m.-11a.m.	3a.m.-7a.m.	3p.m.-7p.m.

These associations work broadly speaking as follows: the energy of the phase is often unbalanced by its associations, but may show symptoms of them also. Thus Fire problems might occur between 11 a.m. and 3 p.m. and show, or be worsened by, a desire for burnt food. They might appear as someone who laughed overmuch; and laughing might be dangerous! They may occur in summer or when it is hot, or be aggravated in heated conditions.

Time — these are the times allocated by the law of midday-midnight: the 24-hour clock, which shows the time when one form of qi reaches a particular place in the meridian cycle — not to be confused with the times indicated by the four-phase cycle.

FURTHER READING

Chinese Medicine
T. J. Kaptchuk, *The Webb that has no Weaver* (St. Martin's Press, U.S., 1983).
K. Matsumoto and S. Birch, *Five Eelments and Ten Stems* (Paradigm Pubns., U.S., 1983).
M. Porkert, *The Theoretical Foundations of Chinese Medicine* (M.I.T. Press, 1978).

Astrology
R. Hand, *Horoscope Symbols* (Para Research, U.S., 1981).
Mayo, *Planets and Human Behaviour* (L. N. Fowler, 1972).
C. E. O. Carter, *The Astrological Aspects* (L. N. Fowler, 1960).

GLOSSARY

Benefic   Classical description of the nature of Venus and Jupiter, respectively lesser and greater benefics.

Chou   (Spelt *jiao* or *jou* in some texts.) Pronounced *choo*. A burning space, place of heat, or energy area.

Upper chou: area of the chest above the diaphragm, containing lungs, pericardium and heart, stores a pure form of qi, likened to 'mist'. This form of qi is essential, like breathing, for a clear head, good circulation and for action. Certain states of mental disequilibrium are caused by what is called 'mist obstructing the orifices of the heart'.

Middle chou: approximately the space below the diaphragm and above the umbilicus. Mainly connected with digestion and sorting of food and liquid. Energy derived from these sources becomes Blood after being processed in the upper chou. The middle chou is like a 'muddy pool'.

Lower chou: the abdominal space roughly inferior to the umbilicus, said to contain the intestines, the uterus, kidney and bladder. It contains our long-term energy resources, and is like a drain or aqueduct.

Cycles   Several cycles are discussed in this book. The four-and five-phase cycles are discribed in Chapter 1. The five-phase, or *sheng* cycle (Diagram 7) is the source of understanding one way in which energy moves to nourish each pair of coupled *zangfu* in turn.

The *ke* or *ko* cycle (Diagram 8) is a controlling cycle. Thus weak Kidney qi allows Heart energy to become overactive, leading perhaps to panic and hysteria with palpitations. The *wu* cycle is the reverse of the *ke* cycle, so moves in the direction Lung-Heart-Kidney-Spleen-Liver-Lung. If Heart energy becomes too powerful there may be a reciprocal change in the Kidney energy.

Division   The *Six Divisions* (three yang and three yin) are a concept to explain the progress of some diseases. Syndromes of the six divisions are reflections of pathological changes in the meridians and zangfu organs when invaded by pathogenic factors. The three yang syndromes, for example, are based on pathological changes of the *fu* organs; e.g. the fu organ of the 'Foot Tai Yang' is Bladder, which has a close relationship with skin and hair. So Tai Yang syndromes occur where pathological factors are at a superficial level of the body energy, and where there is a dysfunction of the Bladder in dividing 'clear' and 'turbid' fluids, and in discharging urine.

(In Western medicine, the function of separating the fluids is given to the kidney organ. In giving this function to the Bladder, traditional Chinese medicine shows again the mistake of confusing an energy orb with an underlying organ. No such mistake occurs in Chinese writing, because the Bladder meridian is known as the Foot Tai Yang, or Foot Great Yang. This distinguishes it from the Hand Tai Yang, or Hand Great Yang which in the West is called the Small Intestine meridian.

In order to keep to a minimum the number of Chinese terms, the energy orbs have been called Bladder, Small Intestine etc. The disadvantage of this becomes apparent when further concepts, such as the Six Divisions, are mentioned.)

Extra Meridians   Like reservoirs in a giant hydroelectric and irrigation scheme, the Eight Extra Meridians can be used as sources of both Blood and qi, absorbing excess and releasing reserves according to need. They have important duties in connection with protection and growth. Only two of the Eight Extra Meridians, Du Mo and Ren Mo, have their own points. The other six borrow points from other meridians, forming a detailed lattice of energy interconnections. Besides these eight, there are many other important meridians, not mentioned in this book.

Fu

Hollow organ. The six ordinary fu are Small Intestine, Stomach, Large Intestine, Bladder, Gall Bladder and Three Heater, or Three Chou, the latter being a collection of some of the functions shared by other zangfu within the body cavity. (See under *Chou* above.) Each fu is linked to a zang organ (see below). In general the six ordinary fu are empty organs which receive and digest food, absorb nutrient substances and transmit and excrete waste. In addition, there are other 'extraordinary fu', not coupled directly with the zang organs. These are the brain, uterus, vascular system, bone-marrow and gall bladder. Gall bladder appears twice; it has a dual role.

Houses

Twelve sectors of the birth chart; each traditionally allocated to a sphere of life. They are counted anti-clockwise, the first house beginning with its cusp or entry point on the Ascendant. There are many different house systems. Apart from passing references, the use of houses is avoided in this book.

Jing

Essence: the substance arising from the parental bond; the basis of our inborn constitution.

Jinye

'Impure' organic body fluids. For example, milk from the mammary glands, tears, saliva, mucus, sweat and moisture coating the lungs. Urine is considered to be a waste fluid.

Malefic

Classical description of the nature of Mars and Saturn, respectively the lesser and greater malefics.

Meridian

A channel or pathway connecting energy centres and points, used in acupuncture.

Moss	Tongue coating. The condition, colour and moss of the tongue are important diagnostically.
P'o	Hereditary instincts and programming.
Principles	The *Eight Principles*, like the five phases, are ways of judging a disease. The eight principles are a more detailed breakdown of yin and yang.

yin: Cold, interior, deficient.
yang: hot, exterior, excess.

E.g. A disease that makes a patient cold and weak and attacks deep inside may be said to be yin. Many conditions are mixed as, for instance, where a patient is chilly but dislikes heat.

Broadly speaking, in practice, the Eight Principles determine whether to tonify or to disperse energy, whereas the Five Phases show which energy system needs attention.

Progressions	The consecutive positions of a planet in the period before or after birth, measured according to certain rules. Thus 'secondary' progressions measure the position of each planet on consecutive days after birth on the principal that movement during each 24 hours represents, symbolically, each consecutive year of life: a 'day for a year'.
Pulse	The pulse in traditional Chinese medicine is a more sophisticated diagnostic tool than its Western counterpart. For example, on each wrist there are three positions, each having up to three depths where separate information is gathered. Taking both wrists together there are therefore between twelve and eighteen positions (depending on which system is used) for assessing the pulse. Each of these positions can have different pulse qualities, and twenty-nine pulse qualities are discussed in the literature. Each pulse quality denotes a number of possible energetic states. For instance, a slow pulse usually suggests either Cold, yang deficiency, or injury of the Heart, whereas a fast pulse means either Heat, much yang qi, empty yin, shock, Blood qi deficiency or/and sometimes Empty yang

producing Empty Cold, allowing qi to escape. Others factors confirm the diagnosis.

Qi Pronounced *chee*. Energy, vitality. There are many different kinds of qi.

Shen The Spirit, manifested in vitality, awareness and mental ability.

Transit The position of a planet in the sky at a particular moment. For example, transiting Uranus at the time of an accident.

Wei qi Defensive energy, mobilized by Liver, but disposed by Lung. Closely connected with opening and closing the pores of the skin.

Zang Solid organ. The six zang organs are Heart, Spleen, Lung, Kidney, Liver and Pericardium. They exist to manufacture and store qi, Blood and Body fluid.

Zangfu There is a clear relationship between coupled organs of zang and fu. The activity of any zang or fu cannot be exactly related to its Western equivalent.

ASTROLOGICAL SYMBOLS

Planets
☉	Sun	♄	Saturn
☽	Moon	♅	Uranus
☿	Mercury	♆	Neptune
♀	Venus	♇	Pluto
♂	Mars	☊	Dragon's Head (North Node)
♃	Jupiter	☋	Dragon's Tail (South Node)

Signs
♈	Aries	♎	Libra
♉	Taurus	♏	Scorpio
♊	Gemini	♐	Sagittarius
♋	Cancer	♑	Capricorn
♌	Leo	♒	Aquarius
♍	Virgo	♓	Pisces

Angles
A   Ascendant
D   Descendant
M   Medium coeli
I   Imum coeli

Aspects
☌	Conjunct	Distance between planets =	0°
☍	Opposite	=	180°
□	Square	=	90°
∠	Semisquare	=	45°
⚼	Sesquiquadrate	=	135°

Δ	Trine	= 120°
★	Sextile	= 60°
T	Transiting	
P	Progressed	

In the charts in this book, all planets and angles are shown to the nearest ½ degree.

INDEX